English and Reflective Writing Skills in Medicine

English and Reflective Writing Skills in Medicine

A GUIDE FOR MEDICAL STUDENTS AND DOCTORS

CLIVE HANDLER

BSc (Hons), MB BS, MD, MRCP, FACC, FESC
Consultant Cardiologist,
Consultant in Pulmonary Hypertension, Royal Free Hospital
Honorary Senior Lecturer, Division of Medicine,
UCL Medical School
Honorary Consultant Cardiologist,
Guy's and St Thomas' Hospitals

CHARLOTTE HANDLER

BA (Hons)
Teacher of English,
JFS School, London

and

DEBORAH GILL

MB BS, MRCGP, MMEd, FHEA
Senior Lecturer in Medical Education,
Division of Medical Education, UCL Medical School

Foreword by

PROFESSOR SIR JOHN TOOKE

FRCP, FMedSci
Head, UCL School of Life and Medical Sciences
and UCL Medical School

Radcliffe Publishing
London • New York

Radcliffe Publishing Ltd
33–41 Dallington Street
London
EC1V 0BB
United Kingdom

www.radcliffepublishing.com

Electronic catalogue and worldwide online ordering facility.

British Library Cataloguing in Publication Data

A catalogue record for this book is available from the British Library.

ISBN-13: 978 184619 462 7

The paper used for the text pages of this book is FSC® certified. FSC (The Forest Stewardship Council®) is an international network to promote responsible management of the world's forests.

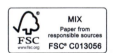

MIX
Paper from
responsible sources
FSC® C013056

Typeset by Pindar NZ, Auckland, New Zealand
Printed and bound by TJI Digital, Padstow, Cornwall, UK

Contents

Foreword

The UK consensus statement on the contemporary role of the doctor states: "All doctors must be demonstrably committed to reflective practice, monitoring their contribution and working continually to improve their own and their team's performance". Enhancing one's own contribution requires the capacity to reflect on one's performance as the foundation for improvement. Committing that process to the written word encourages rigour and provides a record of self-development, the latter an increasingly important requirement. Against this background, this book is a timely source of clarity and stimulus for the development of effective reflective writing that will aid medical students, doctors in training and established practitioners wishing to hone their skills. Rather than "model answers" the book uses the device of revealing the uncorrected (anonymous) reflective essays from third-year medical students to highlight the good and the not so good and where change is necessary.

In health there is much emphasis on good communication skills, which usually focus on oral and non-verbal elements. The written record (the illegibility of which is stereotypical of doctors) is equally important, with good-quality English being the critical component. If we heed the lessons herein, this book will make an important contribution to the quality of care.

Professor Sir John Tooke, FRCP, FMedSci
Head, UCL School of Life and Medical Sciences
and UCL Medical School
February 2011

Preface

Most medical students do not study English or other essay-based subjects at A Level and, by nature and education, are scientists rather than craftsmen in English Literature and creative writing. Generally, their skills in science tend to be more developed than their creative writing skills. Writing good, concise, well-structured and correctly spelled and punctuated English has always been an essential part of effective communication among doctors, other healthcare professionals and patients, and is becoming increasingly important. Good communication underpins good clinical practice. In many respects, the care a doctor takes in their written communication reflects the care taken in clinical and organisational matters.

The ability to write good English is essential for applicants to medical school when they write their personal statement, a key component of the application. It provides a valuable insight into the abilities of the applicant. A poorly written statement is not a good start. The essay section of the BioMedical Admissions Test (BMAT), required by some universities, constitutes a significant element in the overall score. At UCL (University College London), the essay is part of the interview; applicants are given the essay they wrote in the examination to discuss during the interview. A well-written essay is a major advantage for the applicant. A less than satisfactory essay is a stumbling block.

Once accepted into medical school, good written English remains essential. Reflective writing is an established and increasingly important educational discipline in many of the UK medical schools. Students are required to submit essays or reports during their clinical course and, not surprisingly perhaps, many find this challenging.

Reflecting on various educational experiences (clinical encounters, practical procedures, conferences and self-directed learning) are an integral part of continuing professional development for doctors, nurses and other healthcare professionals. They are also an important component of job applications and appraisals and a central aspect of plans for revalidation.

Reflective writing is difficult because by its very nature it is highly personal, subjective and often emotive. It demands several characteristics: sensitivity, sensibility, emotional intelligence, insight and the ability to be self-critical and to provide a balanced analysis of an important clinical encounter or event. People feel differently about the same event; we all learn different things from the same experience. The author has to be honest enough to disclose to the reader what they felt at the time and later, and how, on reflection, they could have performed better and what they have learned from the event. Reflection aims to help doctors perform better the next time they are faced with a similar situation. Each stage of the reflective process is challenging, particularly when describing what has been learned, because this implies that the author was unaware or ignorant of this aspect before the event. This should not be a cause of embarrassment. The purpose of reflective practice is self-education. Most young people, and, indeed, many older people, feel uncomfortable disclosing their personal frailties. This often becomes less uncomfortable as we develop and gain more experience of human nature, and learn about similar or even worse frailties in others!

The skills to express yourself clearly and keep your reader interested are fundamentally important in reflective writing. This demands a good grasp of the fundamentals of English grammar and writing: these are the tools of expression. When you write you must have a clear idea of what you want to tell your readers. The first few lines should transport them to the scene so they appreciate the situation you were in at the time of writing and, if relevant, the people who were with you. You have to explain how you felt at the time and later, what you think you did well and what did not go well and how you think others might have viewed your performance. Importantly, what were your conclusions, what did you learn and how will this affect what you do next time? Your reader might disagree with your analysis of the situation and this is because we all see events differently; an event you find disturbing or impressive may not have a similar effect on someone else.

We have written this book to help medical students, doctors and other healthcare professionals understand what reflection is, to point out the attributes of a satisfactory or good reflective essay, and what makes a reflective essay unsatisfactory. We also focus on the quality of the English writing, which we feel is at least as important as the quality of the reflection, and we provide guidelines on how to write satisfactory English. This has been a difficult task for us because there is no "correct" or approved way to write a good reflective essay, although there are certain fundamentals. Whilst spotting "good" and "bad" written English is relatively easy, marking essays with a summative comment is more challenging. Each essay can contain a multitude of different types of problems. Marking is rarely a clear-cut, categorical process. We have not attempted to comment on every error in each essay. For the purposes of this book, we have focused and commented on the most prominent problem areas in each essay. We have selected a range of essays that we hope illustrate both good and unsatisfactory standards of English writing. Writing is like other disciplines; interest in producing a good piece, practice, revision and refinement will improve your skills. There is a general consensus on what constitutes a good reflective essay and we hope that this short book will go some way to showing what would be considered by most tutors to fit the bill.

We invited our third-year clinical students to submit their essays for publication, informing them that we wanted to publish their uncorrected essays, which we thought highlighted both satisfactory and unsatisfactory examples of reflection and English. The essays are published anonymously and in a random order. We publish the names of the contributing authors who wished their names to be published and we are very grateful to them. They have exposed their own successes and failures to help you to grasp what might be required of you as a professional or developing professional when asked to write a reflective piece. We, along with our students, have learned and continue to learn about reflection and strive to improve the quality of our written English. We hope that our readers will be similarly inspired by these essays and our comments and will find reflective practice an enjoyable and useful part of their professional work.

Clive Handler, Charlotte Handler, Deborah Gill
February 2011

About the authors

Clive Handler is a consultant cardiologist. He is consultant in pulmonary hypertension at the National Pulmonary Hypertension Unit, the Royal Free Hospital; Honorary Consultant Cardiologist, Guy's and St Thomas' NHS Foundation Trust; and Honorary Senior Lecturer, Division of Medicine, UCL Medical School. He edited *Guy's Hospital: 250 Years*; co-authored *Cardiology in Primary Care, Management of Cardiac Problems in Primary Care* and *Preventing Cardiovascular Disease in Primary Care* (all published by Radcliffe Publishing); co-edited *Classic Papers in Coronary Angioplasty, Vascular Complications of Human Disease: Mechanisms and Consequences* and *Advances in Vascular Medicine*; and co-authored *Living with Coronary Disease* (Springer) and *Pulmonary Arterial Hypertension: The Facts* and *The Oxford Handbook of Pulmonary Hypertension* (Oxford University Press). He is the author of numerous papers in general medicine and cardiology.

Charlotte Handler was educated at North London Collegiate School. She read English at the University of Bristol and then completed the Postgraduate Certificate in Education at Middlesex University, specialising in English at secondary school level. Charlotte teaches English Literature and Language at the JFS school in London.

Deborah Gill is a senior clinical academic in medical education and director of the Academic Centre for Medical Education at UCL Medical School. She has a broad portfolio of academic roles in both undergraduate and postgraduate education and training. As Sub-Dean for curriculum development and innovation she is lead for the personal and professional development aspects of the undergraduate programme, including reflective practice. She is involved in faculty development for educators with a large number of National Health Service trusts, the London and Eastern deaneries, the Royal College of Physicians and the General Medical Council. She is a member of the ASME (Association for the Study of Medical Education) Council and a peer reviewer for a number of education journals. Her research interests include support of novices (both doctors and teachers), portfolio learning and personal and professional development.

List of contributors

We are grateful to the following students at UCL (University College London) who kindly allowed us to use their essays, "warts and all", to help others to learn about reflective writing. Without their generosity, this book would not exist.

- Omid Alavijeh
- Alison Berner
- Anna Burford
- Neha Desai
- Sarah Donaldson
- Jasmine Ehsanulla
- Aidan Fullbrook
- Beth Goulden
- George Hadjivassiliou
- Quentin Huys
- Natasha Hyder
- Yasmin Kamheih
- Aga Reza Ali Khan
- Shamim Lakha
- Vincent Lam
- Cara Lewis
- Yik Man
- Farwah Medhi
- Kumaran Mylvaganam
- Aniket Nadgir
- Arjuna Nagendran
- Brenavan Natarajan
- Zahra Rajput
- Mohsen Raza
- Savasti Salie
- Benjamin Shaw
- Alexandra Shepherd
- Sam Shribman
- Harjah Siraj
- Amanda Smith

- Vera Strusevich
- Ayeshah Waheed
- Christopher Wilding
- Alice Wilson

CHAPTER 1

Reflective practice and written reflection in medicine

In this chapter we outline what "reflection" in education has come to mean and why reflective practice is seen as important in education for the professions. We look at reflective writing, outlining when and why it is used in medicine and medical education and what constitutes good reflective writing. We have used the current guidance for medical students at UCL Medical School as a framework for answering questions such as: What is a good incident to use as a focus for reflection? What does a good piece of reflective writing look like? What framework should I use to construct a good piece of reflective writing?

As reflective practice tutors who regularly read reflective pieces and give students what we hope is useful feedback, we have also made suggestions about what constitutes useful feedback for students as they develop this complex cognitive and expressive skill, and we highlight the debate concerning whether you can "mark" reflection.

By exploring these areas we hope to draw the reader's attention to the fact that reflection, reflective practice and reflective writing are difficult concepts to define clearly for both teachers and learners, and that this lack of clarity sometimes leads teachers to adopt loose definitions and provide vague guidance, leaving learners struggling to understand the usefulness of reflective activities or what is required of them.

Finally, throughout the chapter we offer some frameworks for novices that may be helpful in understanding the purpose of reflective practice so they can improve their attempts at reflection and reflective writing.

WHAT IS REFLECTION?

In the last few decades, reflection and reflective practice have become an accepted organising framework for professional preparation and practice (Boud and Walker

1998) and consequently activities to encourage the development of reflective abilities have become established components of contemporary education for all professions, including medicine. But what exactly is reflection?

Definitions of reflection in the context of learning are plentiful in the literature; however, the term "reflection" may be used to refer to a wide array of cognitively and philosophically distinct methods and attitudes (Van Manen 1995).

In medical education a frequently used definition is one by Moon that suggests:

> Reflection is a form of mental processing . . . that we use to fulfil a purpose or to achieve some anticipated outcome. It is applied to relatively complicated or unstructured ideas for which there is not an obvious solution and is largely based on the further processing of knowledge and understanding and possibly emotions that we already possess.
>
> (Moon 1999: 5)

Other useful definitions refer to reflection as when individuals purposefully explore experiences that bring about changes in perspective and understanding:

> Reflection refers to all those intellectual and affective activities in which individuals engage to explore their experiences in order to lead to new understandings and appreciations.
>
> (Boud *et al.* 1985: 19)

> The process of internally examining and exploring an issue of concern, triggered by an experience, which creates and clarifies meaning in terms of self, and which results in a changed conceptual perspective.
>
> (Boyd and Fales 1983: 99)

The idea of reflection as a contributor to the enhancement of practice has its foundations in the work of John Dewey (1933). He first described reflection in terms of "thinking about thinking". Dewey wrote extensively about "reflective thought"; thoughts and reflections provoked by an event that arouses a state of doubt, perplexity or uncertainty, and that leads the individual to search for possible explanations or solutions.

Donald Schön (1983) coined the term "reflective practice" and argued that professionals in their everyday practice face unique and complex situations that are unsolvable by the "technical rationality" approaches that had been the dominant paradigm in professional and scientific learning since the nineteenth century. Schön suggests professional practice is largely based upon tacit knowledge (knowing-in-action) and that professionals increasingly engage in "reflective conversation with the situation" as practice becomes stable. Schön also proposes that practitioners go on to reflect *on* action; a more extended and sustained review that occurs later on, after the event, and provides opportunities to learn from the earlier decision-making process or reflection-in-action (1987).

REFLECTIVE PRACTICE AND EDUCATION FOR THE HEALTH PROFESSIONS

It is generally assumed that reflective practice, and thus the notion of the preparedness of health professionals to think critically and to engage themselves in reflection upon their professional activities, will contribute to the improvement of their performance (Mamede and Schmidt 2004). The result of this assumption is that reflection is regarded as a core skill in professional competence (Epstein and Hundert 2002). However, it has been argued that reflective theory and practice has little irrefutable evidence of effectiveness in the health professions (Burton 2000).

The emphasis by the General Medical Council (GMC) for doctors to develop and practise reflection suggests the fundamental aim of reflection and reflective practice within medical education is to ultimately improve patient care (GMC 2006).

Undergraduate medical education has thus, unsurprisingly, embraced a reflective practice component. However, as Schön postulates, being critically self-aware is an acquired skill and cognitive restructuring of knowledge comes with experience and is characteristically an expert act (Ericsson and Charness 1994). It is unsurprising, therefore, that medical students find the practice of reflection difficult and struggle with creating meaning from the process.

As educators we are often unclear as to what we are asking students to do when they undertake reflective practice, and to what end. The fact that students often entitle their written work "reflective practise", as opposed to the term *reflective practice* used by their teachers and curriculum designers, is an interesting one: do they not know the difference between the spelling of the word as a noun as opposed to a verb? Or are they seeing this as *practising* a skill, much like one might practise taking blood, rather than as a distinct activity or behaviour in itself, purposeful in its own right?

It is worth noting that reflective practice has been adopted in the health professions in modern times beyond its original intention of the examination of personal experience to be used as an aspect of "proof" of professional development; one of the many facets of modern medicine whereby the actions of professionals have become "rooted in the public and political as well as the private and personal" (Bolton 2001: 5). This has some implications for the "honesty" of reflections, limiting what practitioners of all levels of experience are prepared to share either verbally or in writing.

In the process of reflection, individuals use a number of personal and cognitive skills: self-awareness, description, critical analysis and evaluation; it is important that we acknowledge the difficulty most learners will have in being reflective in the way we expect them to be, and in articulating this new way of thinking.

A practical and explanatory description of purposeful reflection that could usefully be shared with novices might include the following.

Acknowledging the purpose
➤ A deliberate act where an individual explores their experiences and becomes more "mindful" of an event, in order to arrive at new understandings and appreciations.

Selecting an event
➤ Choosing an incident that has been significant to you: preferably one that remains "unsorted" to some extent and where deeper "reflection-on-action" may help you to understand your own motives and actions and the motives and actions of others. This does not have to be a major incident or an alarming event: simply an episode that sticks in the mind and cannot easily be put aside.

Description
➤ Giving a description that provides enough of the detail that makes the incident worthy of reflection but recognising this is the first stepping stone to the reflection: it is not the whole act.

Critically analysing the description
➤ Being honest in how the event affected you as an individual and the impact that may have had within the event.
➤ Stepping back and exploring and challenging assumptions and conclusions: considering alternative explanations of events than those initially reached.
➤ Being self-aware, accepting that there may be other ways of thinking about your actions or omissions.

Evaluation
➤ To develop new perspectives on the event and to acknowledge what you have learned from it and how you might behave or think differently in the future. This needs to be more than a bland statement such as "next time I will be more assertive": it needs to consider what you might do or say and any difficulties you may have in carrying out the planned actions.

REFLECTIVE WRITING

If developing the skills of a reflective practitioner is about thinking about action both in the moment and after the event, then reflective writing has the potential to extend this reflection. It is a way of rethinking or reframing the experience (Feest and Forbes 2007) that may lead to deeper levels of understanding and the potential for meaningful personal and professional growth.

Hatton and Smith (1995) suggest a hierarchy for describing the levels of reflection in written work.
➤ **Descriptive writing:** Description of events or literature reports. No discussion beyond description. The writing is considered not to show evidence of reflection.
➤ **Descriptive reflection:** Basically description, but some evidence of deeper consideration. No real evidence of the notion of alternative viewpoints in use.
➤ **Dialogic reflection:** Writing suggests "stepping back" from events and actions leads to different level of discourse. Sense of "mulling about" and exploration of personal role in events and actions. Consideration of the qualities of

judgements and possible alternative explanations. Reflection is analytical or integrative, linking factors and perspectives.

➤ **Critical reflection:** In addition, shows evidence that the learner is aware that actions and events may be "located within and explicable by multiple perspectives, but are located in and influenced by multiple and socio-political contexts" (1995: 49).

In the context of professional learning and professional development it is *critical reflection* that is expected; the ability of the professional (or professional in training) to step back from events, to explore what has happened by exploring their reflections-in-action and their reflections-on-action. It involves recognising theirs is only one of a range of possible interpretations, and an attempt to make some sense of things that enables them to see themselves and their actions more clearly. Simply describing events and making unsophisticated comments such as "I will not do that in the future" or "doctors should/shouldn't do this" does not represent the level of reflection that reflective practitioners should be aiming for.

Novices may like to use a framework, particularly if they are new to reflective writing or if reflecting or writing does not come naturally. There are a number of frameworks that can help those who are reflecting to make the process more purposeful and to get to this deeper level of reflection.

At UCL Medical School we offer, and discuss with our students, the following framework to guide them as they begin to undertake reflective writing: "Structured Debriefing" from *Learning by Doing* (Gibbs 1988), based on Kolb's experiential learning cycle. The framework consists of several structured steps:

➤ Description: What is the stimulant for reflection (incident, event, idea)? What are you going to reflect on?

➤ Feelings: What were your reactions and feelings?

➤ Evaluation: What was good and bad about the experience? (make value judgements)

➤ Analysis: What sense can you make of the situation? (bring in ideas from outside the experience to help you. What was really going on?)

➤ Conclusions (general): What can be concluded, in a general sense, from these experiences and the analyses you have undertaken?

➤ Conclusions (specific): What can be concluded about your own specific, unique personal situation or ways of working?

➤ Personal action plans: What are you going to do differently in this type of situation next time? What steps are you going to take on the basis of what you have learned?

As highlighted, documented reflective practice has become a requirement to "prove" a certain level of professionalism; consequently, reflective writing is often a core aspect of the personal and professional development domain of the undergraduate medical course, often in the form of entries into a portfolio. The purpose of a portfolio in vocational courses such as medicine has become to allow the development *and assessment* of aspects of professional behaviour and learning. A medical undergraduate portfolio is, therefore, a hybrid beast: *personal* in the process of encouraging the process of reflection but *public* in the need to demonstrate professional behaviour. Because of this, many written reflective pieces are often "far from reflection and indeed . . . merely diary entries describing an event or activity" (Woodward 1998: 417). There is little doubt that such forced reflection raises moral and practical issues and often results in learners producing superficial or guarded reflections. Whether reflective practice "can be a required component of a course and still retain validity as genuine reflection" (Hobbs 2007: 406) is questionable.

WHAT IS A GOOD THING TO REFLECT UPON?

Novices often ask this question and the simple answer is any experience that has made you stop and think. Whilst we are mindful of what we do most of the time, sometimes we challenge and question ourselves more fully, or look for new and improved ways of working, when things don't go to plan. Often the stimulus is something that is not easily "sortable" by simple, in-the-moment thinking on our feet.

On the whole the best professional growth comes from exploring ourselves and our own actions. However, it is possible to write a reflective piece about the actions of someone else; so long as we analyse this in the context of the effect it had on us. The following are some suggestions of areas and experiences that can generate good critical reflections.

About a patient
➤ A patient happy or unhappy with their treatment by you or others.
➤ A question of confidentiality, consent or inappropriate risk.
➤ Doing something for the first time.
➤ Communicating with older or frail people.
➤ Consultations involving more than one person (for example, a relative).
➤ Sudden death or deterioration.

About you
➤ An aspect of a patient encounter that revealed gaps in your knowledge or skills.
➤ An event that caused you anxiety or enjoyment.
➤ An aspect of care that left you surprised, puzzled or confused.
➤ A patient that challenged your assumptions or whose actions are at odds with your personal beliefs and values.

About the team
➤ When you feel an aspect of the treatment or management is wrong.
➤ A dysfunctional team that affects patient outcomes or experiences.
➤ The actions of the team under pressure.

Good medical practice
➤ Times when you have exhibited good medical practice or found yourself in a situation that may be at odds with good medical practice.
➤ Times when you have seen medical practice or behaviour that may be at odds with good medical practice.

MARKING AND GIVING FEEDBACK ON REFLECTIVE WRITING

Most professionals develop reflective skills; assisted by the processes of appraisal and professional development planning they strive for improvement in their practice, they challenge and question themselves, and they look for new and improved ways of working. Helping those who are beginning to develop their professional skills involves guiding them in these processes, and giving constructive feedback with the aim of helping them to gain insight:

> Giving feedback is not just to provide a judgement or evaluation. It is to provide insight. Without insight into their own limitations trainees cannot progress or resolve difficulties.
>
> (King 1999: S2)

As previously noted, the process of reflection involves description, critical analysis, self-awareness and evaluation. In addition to this, reflective writing requires further skills: the ability to articulate these thought processes clearly and concisely and the use of good written English. What constitutes useful feedback for students as they develop this complex cognitive and expressive skill is not straightforward.

The most important issue for teachers working in the domain of reflective practice is to recognise that helping a learner to develop as a reflective practitioner is firmly within the "education as transformation of the person" approach, as opposed to the "education as transmission of material" approach. This is not a recipe that can be followed and will always be perfect, nor is there only one way to be reflective.

Whilst most professionals develop good reflective skills, not all professionals develop good writing skills. Medicine has always been a world where you are judged by what you have written, for example in notes and letters. Today, with the incorporation of reflective writing into portfolios, application forms, appraisals and revalidations, impressions generated by what you have written count for even more.

Feedback needs to be sensitive but must challenge as well as support, encouraging the student to develop insight into actions and reactions to further develop their reflection and to accept comments on the use of English as constructive rather than critical. Often reflection involves descriptions of actions or inactions of self or others and it is important for those giving feedback to minimise judgmental comments, instead probing for explanations and highlighting effect, rather than making assumptions about intent.

As tutors regularly giving feedback to novices in this domain, the most common areas on which we give feedback are getting bogged down with description of the event rather than reflection, limiting the reflection to descriptive reflection (*see* levels of reflective writing section above), the absence of a well-thought-through consideration of plans for future action, and either careless attention to the use of English or significant difficulties in the correct use of written English.

Whilst the content of reflective writing is obviously very important, the quality of the writing and writing style is also key. From our experience, and as you will see in many of the examples in the book, a large number of students are let down by their written English. Poor grammar, spelling, punctuation and sentence and paragraph cohesion regularly flaw countless submissions every year.

Grammatical perfection is difficult to attain, indeed there is no one set of easy rules to follow that guarantee success every time, nor one "correct way" to do things, so it is important to not be too pedantic about split infinitives or the Oxford comma. However, there are some general rules that make *reading for understanding* easier and it is important for students to be told about *what* and *how* they can improve next time in their use of English, particularly if English is not their first language. As the American author Nathaniel Hawthorne reminds us: "Easy reading is damn hard writing", so as a tutor if you find something a joy to read, remember to congratulate the author on this aspect of their reflective writing as well as the content of the reflection.

ASSESSING REFLECTIVE WRITING

Since the introduction of written reflection in the development of professional practice, there has been debate about whether reflective writing can or should be marked. In a competency-driven education culture there is a tendency to reduce all learning to a tick-box exercise confirming whether or not mastery of a skill has been acquired. Professional development and reflective practice challenge this approach. Difficulties such as poor inter-rater reliability and difficulty in applying conventional assessment criteria to this complex and highly personal activity lead to poor reliability (Pitts *et al.* 2002), and provide an argument against formally assessing reflection. Others suggest that assessment is necessary to encourage student engagement (Driessen *et al.* 2005).

At UCL (University College London) after much debate we have chosen to concentrate on feedback and to limit possible marks to "suitable for submission to portfolio" or "not suitable for submission". If students have failed to engage fully in the process or to grasp the activity, they are given an opportunity to incorporate the feedback and rewrite the submission.

In conclusion reflective practice is a difficult concept to clearly define for both teachers and learners. This lack of clarity may lead teachers to loosely define the process and thus not clearly advocate either the utility or the purpose of activities based around developing reflective practice. Equally, whilst the notion of reflecting on practice seems highly valid to an experienced professional, it might be expected that undergraduates may question the usefulness of the activity, failing to see the purpose of critical self-awareness in their learning. Novices may find the process difficult and may see a separate deliberate processing phase (Boud *et al.* 1985) as unnecessary in their learning from experience. For all of these reasons, together with the public nature of professional reflections, they may develop a rather superficial and cautious "going through the motions" approach to such learning activities. The role of the teacher is to encourage brave and meaningful reflection and to ensure feedback is mindful of both practice and writing.

BIBLIOGRAPHY

Bolton G. *Reflective Practice: writing and professional development.* London: Sage Publications; 2001.

Boud D, Keogh R, Walker D, editors. *Reflection: turning experience into learning.* London: Kogan Page; 1985.

Boud D, Walker D. Promoting reflection in professional courses: the challenge of context. *Stud High Educ.* 1998; **23**(2): 191–206.

Boyd E, Fales A. Reflective learning: the key to learning from experience. *J Humanist Psychol.* 1983; **23**(2): 99–117.

Burton AJ. Reflection: nursing's practice and education panacea? *J Adv Nurs.* 2000; **31**(5): 1009–17.

Davis MH, Friedman Ben-David M, Harden RM, *et al.* Portfolio assessment in medical students' final examinations. *Med Teach.* 2001; **23**(4): 357–66.

Dewey J. *How We Think.* Boston, MA: DC Heath; 1933.

Driessen EW, van Tartwijk J, Overeem K, *et al.* Conditions for successful reflective use of portfolios in undergraduate medical education. *Med Educ.* 2005; **39**(12): 1230–5.

Epstein RM, Hundert EM. Defining and assessing professional competence. *JAMA.* 2002; **287**(2): 226–35.

Ericsson KA, Charness N. Expert performance: its structure and acquisition. *Am Psychol.* 1994; **49**(8): 725–46.

Feest K, Forbes K. *Today's Students, Tomorrow's Doctors: reflections from the wards.* Oxford: Radcliffe Publishing; 2007.

Gibbs G. *Learning by Doing: a guide to teaching and learning methods.* Oxford: Further Educational Unit; 1988.

GMC (General Medical Council). *Good Medical Practice.* 4th ed. London: GMC; 2006.

Hatton N, Smith D. Reflection in teacher education: towards definition and implementation. *Teach Teach Educ.* 1995; **11**(1): 33–49.

Hobbs V. Faking it or hating it: can reflective practice be forced? *Reflective Practice.* 2007; **8**(3): 405–17.

King J. Giving feedback. *BMJ.* 1999; **318**(2): 7200.

Mamede S, Schmidt HG. The structure of reflective practice in medicine. *Med Educ.* 2004; **38**(12):1302–8.

Moon J. *Learning Journals: a handbook for academics, students and professional development.* London: Kogan Page; 1999.

Moon J. *Reflective Writing: some initial guidance for students.* Available at: www.e-radiography.net/projects/relective_writing.htm (accessed 13 January 2011).

Pitts J, Coles C, Thomas P, *et al.* Enhancing reliability in portfolio assessment: discussions between assessors. *Med Teach.* 2002; **24**(2): 197–201.

Schön DA. *The Reflective Practitioner: how professionals think in action.* New York: Basic Books; 1983.

Schön DA. *Educating the Reflective Practitioner.* San Francisco, CA: Jossey-Bass; 1987.

Van Manen M. On the epistemology of reflective practice. *Teachers Teach Theory Pract.* 1995; **1**(1): 33–50.

Woodward H. Reflective journals and portfolios: learning through assessment. *Assess Eval High Educ.* 1998; **23**(4): 415–24.

CHAPTER 2

How to write good English

Words are, of course, the most powerful drug used by mankind . . . Not only do words infect, egotise, narcotise, and paralyse, but they enter into and colour the minutest cells of the brain.

Rudyard Kipling

Rudyard Kipling said these words during a speech he made to the Royal College of Surgeons in London in 1923 to iterate the importance of the spoken and written word to the doctors he addressed. The way Kipling linked words and drugs is significant for doctors, who must approach words with as much, if not more, care than they would drugs; doctors must dedicate as much energy to how they articulate themselves as they do to their clinical practice. Kipling highlighted how words can hold enormous power and have significant consequences. Language must be used appropriately and with care as it can affect the emotional state of another human being. Thus, the importance of clear and appropriate written and verbal communication is paramount in medicine, throughout medical school and beyond.

Although few undergraduate medical degrees feature copious amounts of essay writing, it is essential that young doctors are comfortable with and confident about speaking and writing coherent English. Compulsory course units such as reflective writing and scientific writing demand that students are able to articulate their thoughts in an accurate, succinct and logical manner. Medical tutors and professors often complain that medical students present essays that are ridden with erroneous grammar and spelling, awkward phrasing and rambling sentences that hinder the clarity and quality of their work. This chapter aims to address the issues that medical students seem to encounter when writing essays and advise both those who do and those who do not speak English as a first language of the conventions of good written English.

STRUCTURE: PLANNING, STRUCTURING AND PARAGRAPHS

Planning is integral to writing a good essay. You must order your thoughts and arguments to ensure that your writing is coherent and logical. Your reflection will lack substance without coherence and logic and you will not compel or impress your reader. A sound essay plan will also make your essay a lot easier to write and, although a good plan will take time to devise, it will save you time in the long run as it will ultimately reduce your writing time. An essay plan has the same function as a map: it makes the journey faster and far less stressful. Planning should include a combination of accumulating and sifting through ideas; reflective writing truly does favour quality over quantity. Your writing must be focused and concise, and a tight plan that concentrates only on relevant points will help you achieve this. Keep the plan simple.

When structuring your essay follow the reflective writing guidelines outlined in Chapter 1 that should help you determine the shape and order of your essay. Although there is not an official essay plan for reflective writing, a popular model, based on Kolb's cycle of experiential learning, can be seen in Figure 2.1:

1　Detail of the experience/incident
2　Observations of and reflections upon this experience/ incident
3　General thoughts about the implications of this experience and reflection
4　Detail regarding the implications of these reflections upon future medical practice.

Following this plan or a similar one will ensure that your writing is structured, coherent and, most important, totally focused on reflection and does not simply narrate the situation experienced.

Once you are satisfied that your plan covers the reflective cycle illustrated in

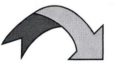

What evidence can you provide to show how you have used this experience to develop your practice and inform your behaviour in professional scenarios?

Identify and describe a professional scenario

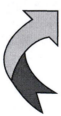

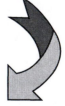

What are the implications for professional practice?

What are the perceived consequences of these behaviours?

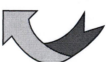

FIGURE 2.1 Kolb's Reflective Cycle

Figure 2.1, the writing process will seem much more straightforward. Focus on one point in each paragraph and ensure that each paragraph has a sense of purpose and links to the next and previous one, thematically and grammatically. Paragraphs function to make your writing more digestible and logical for your reader; paragraph breaks should not be arbitrary and should reflect developments in your essay. There are no concrete rules about paragraph length but your paragraphs should run for at least four sentences. If paragraphs are too brief there is a high risk that the ideas they are presenting will be underdeveloped and therefore unconvincing. On the other hand, if a paragraph takes up more than three-quarters of a page of typed, single-spaced, size 12 font, you may want to reread it and consider whether you could segment it into smaller paragraphs that complement the progression of ideas or a shift in subject matter. Long, overpacked paragraphs can often seem slightly chaotic if too many competing concepts are stuffed into one section.

Once your paragraphs are adequately proportioned, you need to think about linking them together, thematically and grammatically. If you have been following your essay plan, the former should not be difficult. Your reflective writing should systematically take the reader through the events and emotions you experienced; any sudden changes between paragraphs make for a jolted reading experience that will make your reflection seem incoherent. Paragraphs should emerge from and sequence each other and should not appear to spring up from nowhere. The fluidity of your writing will, however, probably be easiest to manage and improve once you have written the essay. It is therefore imperative to ensure that you finish writing your essay well before the deadline and give yourself at least 24 hours to reread, redraft and correct any grammatical or spelling mistakes. At this stage, when you can view your work holistically, it will be easier to identify awkward phrasing or uncomfortable paragraph links and enhance clarity.

SYNTAX AND LENGTH OF SENTENCES

"Syntax" simply refers to sentence construction. Good sentences should be sensibly constructed and logically ordered.

✗ Although we follow a number of patients throughout our clinical practice, from start of treatment to when they are discharged, one of the first patients I saw in clinics I followed at the time thinking that it would have no benefit on my education as I never looked at his charts or notes.

✓ Throughout our clinical practice we follow a number of patients from the start of their treatment to when they are discharged. However, when I encountered one of the first patients I saw in clinics, I was unsure about how educationally beneficial he would be as I never looked at his charts or notes.

A good way to ensure that your written sentences are syntactically correct is to say them aloud and consider whether they sound "right" or slightly awkward. In this respect, good written English is simple: if it doesn't make sense when you say it, it won't make sense when you write it. (If English is not your first language, this may be more difficult so ask a peer to help you out with the proofreading.) Whilst levels of formality may differ between your spoken language and your essay style, syntax won't and reading an essay aloud is often the best way to check that sentences have been well constructed. Sentences should also be grammatically independent: they should make sense on their own. Whilst you might notice incomplete sentences in newspapers and magazines, they are rarely, if ever, appropriate in serious pieces of academic writing. In the following essays and corrections, incomplete sentences are sometimes referred to as "non-sentences".

Example: *Serious threat*. Whilst one could see this type of sentence in a newspaper, it would not be appropriate in academic writing. An improved version could be: It was a serious threat.

THE IMPORTANCE OF USING APPROPRIATE LANGUAGE AND NECESSARY WORDS

People often think that essay markers are impressed by flowery, elaborate and long sentences. This is not the case. The best writing is expressive, succinct and precise. No one benefits from a long-winded, repetitive sentence: you will find it annoying to write and your tutor will find it frustrating to mark. Writing with this economic mindset will also get you into the good habit of distilling your thoughts clearly, which will help you to express various complex situations when you are doctor. If you are ever in doubt about the appropriateness of your language or wording, read the sentence aloud and listen carefully to judge whether it makes sense. Once more you must consider that if you wouldn't say it, you shouldn't write it. If English is not your first language, ask someone who does speak English as a first language to read your work over before you hand it in and ask them whether your wording "sounds right".

USING THE RIGHT TENSE CONSISTENTLY

Many reflective essays dither among the present, past and future tenses in a rather disturbing fashion, hindering the logic and coherence of the writing. Remember to always relate and describe the events you are reflecting on in the *past* tense.

Example: *I saw the patient lying in the ward and was shocked at how she had been treated.*

When you come to the final paragraphs of your essay where you consider the implications of this incident upon future practice, you might want to use the future tense.

Example: *Next time I am in a similar situation, I will act differently.*

You could also use the conditional tense to describe future practice.

Example: *Next time I am in a similar situation, I would act differently.*

THE DANGER OF THE CLICHÉ

Clichés are overused phrases or expressions that have been "used and abused" so many times that they have lost all meaning. Whilst clichés are often used in spoken English, they should never be used in academic writing. If a certain phrase "rings a bell", "sounds like a plan" or seems to be "just the ticket", you are probably using a cliché and it will not be the case of "all's well that ends well". It is "as easy as pie" for clichés to pop up in your writing, whether English is your first language or not, but the key to eliminating these useless and bland phrases from your sentences is to ensure your writing maintains a level of formality and that you read and reread over your essay once you think you have finished. Clichés are not only boring to read but also rarely do justice to your topic: original expressions are inevitably more meaningful and accurate than a collection of overused words.

PERFECTING PUNCTUATION: HOW TO EFFECTIVELY USE COMMAS, SEMICOLONS, COLONS, FULL STOPS, QUESTION MARKS, EXCLAMATION MARKS, SPEECH MARKS, APOSTROPHES, ELLIPSES, DASHES AND BRACKETS

Many people shudder at the word "punctuation" and think of it as a convention that involves the liberal scattering of commas, colons and semicolons over an essay as and when they feel like it for no particular reason. However, punctuation can, quite literally, make or break a sentence. Punctuation should be used as a means of signposting your essay for the reader: you tell them where and when you want them to carry on reading, pause or stop so they can best appreciate what you are telling them about.

Commas indicate where a reader should pause. If you are unsure where to put a comma, read your sentence aloud and note where you would naturally take a breath. You rarely need commas before or after the words "and" or "because" as these words are connectives. Commas can also be used to replace parentheses and can thus be used to subtly separate ideas and clauses within a sentence. These commas are called bracketing commas.

Colons and semicolons are often used interchangeably or avoided altogether, a shame considering each plays a different and important role in sentence construction. **Semicolons** have two functions. They can link two grammatically complete but thematically linked sentences. Semicolons demand a longer pause than commas do.

Example: *It had been a bad day; the ward was full of complaining patients.*

Semicolons can also be used to separate long items in a list.

Example: *The patient was upset about his awful headache; strange purple bruising; intense nausea; and irregular sleeping patterns.*

Colons indicate an even longer pause than a semicolon and are used to introduce a set of ideas. Unlike the semicolon, they are not always followed by a grammatically complete phrase and can be used to introduce a list or a statement that illustrates the first clause.

Example: *The ward was overcrowded and manic: complete chaos.*

Full stops mark the end of a sentence. They are almost always followed by a capital letter, which your computer should do automatically. An essay that solely contains short sentences (and a lot of full stops) can sound both basic and jolted to the reader. An essay that only relies on long, rambling sentences (with few full stops) can sound boring, arrogant and "waffly". The key to using full stops successfully is to remember to vary the length of your sentences throughout your essay. Good pieces of reflective writing will use full stops carefully to vary sentence length, which will add effect, pace and meaning to the writing.

    Question marks are used at the end of a sentence and signify that a question has been asked. You may also use these when reporting questions that were asked during a speech/dialogue you experienced or when you ask yourself a rhetorical question.

Example: *The patient asked me: "Is this treatment really necessary?"*

Example: *Was this the right thing to do? I am still not sure but it made sense at the time.*

Speech marks are used to indicate direct speech and they separate these words from the rest of your sentence.

Example: *"Are you sure?" the Doctor asked me. "Well, almost totally positive", I answered.*

Apostrophes have two main functions: to indicate where letters have been omitted and to show possession.
➤ Apostrophes can abbreviate "cannot" into "can't", "should not" into "shouldn't" and "do not" into "don't". In each case the apostrophe makes up for the letters missed out.
➤ When apostrophes are used to indicate possession they are inserted before the final "s" of a singular noun, for example "the hospital's staff" or "the patient's wishes".
➤ If the noun is a plural, the possessive apostrophe is still inserted before the final "s", for example "the children's ward" or "the staff's uniform".
➤ If the noun ends in an "s" anyway you can insert an apostrophe after the s, for example "the nurses' shouts". You can also insert an apostrophe and add

another "s", for example "St James's Hospital" but the former technique of simply adding a possessive apostrophe after the last "s" is more commonly used.

To use with caution

Exclamation marks should be used with caution in academic writing. They can often make the writing sound too excited and uncontrolled. Whilst they frequent tabloid newspapers and magazines, exclamation marks are rarely appropriate in formal circumstances unless you are reporting speech you overheard. If you want to increase the drama or tension in your writing, just try varying your sentence length and use short, revolutionary statements to depict dramatic moments.

Ellipses should only be used in academic writing to show where you have edited and removed part of a quotation. They should not be used to indicate thoughts fading into oblivion or to create suspense.

Dashes can be used to substitute a colon but, once again, should be used with caution in academic writing. Whilst they are often seen in pieces of media writing, they can look informal and abrupt in academic writing. If you want to signal your reader to pause or if you want to break up ideas within a sentence, use a comma, colon or semicolon as appropriate.

Parentheses or brackets: Brackets are used to insert extra information into a sentence. Whilst they are grammatically acceptable, using brackets excessively (more than one set in each paragraph) can make for a disjointed reading experience as they force the reader to wander from the sentence they are reading. Better are bracketing commas; these are more subtle but no less effective than brackets. Brackets or bracketing commas must be used to separate an idea within a sentence and you can check you have used them correctly by making sure that the sentence would still make sense if the bracketed clause was removed.

WHEN TO USE CAPITAL LETTERS

There are two types of noun: common nouns and proper nouns. Unsurprisingly, common nouns are usually more common in your writing and can be objects, qualities or types of place. Words such as "tube", "bed" and "hospital" are all common nouns. Common nouns do not require capital letters unless they appear at the start of a sentence.

Proper nouns include the names of places and people or certain medical terms and titles. Proper nouns must start with a capital letter. Words such as London, the Royal Free Hospital, Mrs Edwards or Buckingham Palace are proper nouns and must always start with a capital letter, even when they do not begin a sentence. If you are unsure about whether a certain medical term or disease or piece of equipment begins with a capital letter check a textbook or ask a friend. In most such cases, a capital letter will probably not be necessary. Misusing capital letters is a relatively basic grammatical error and tutors can get frustrated if this type of mistake repeatedly appears in your work.

SPELLING

Spelling words correctly is important. If you want to irritate a medical tutor, spell "medicine" or "doctor" incorrectly. Whilst some spelling mistakes can be remedied by a few quick readings over, other errors must be handled in a different way. It is important to never place total faith in the spellcheck on your computer. Although your word processor is programmed to detect and correct spelling errors, it is not able to evaluate the meaning and intentions of your writing. Spellcheck will only pick up on words that are misspelled: it will not detect words that are used inappropriately. For example, when you might recount speaking in a "calm voice" but accidentally type "clam voice", spellcheck will not recognise this error. It is therefore vital that you check your work scrupulously for such "typos" as they will frustrate the meaning of your essay and will also make you seem like a sloppy writer.

Spellcheck will also gloss over correctly spelt but erroneously used homophones (words that sound the same as another word but are spelled differently). Words like "complimentary" and "complementary", "bear" and "bare" and even "where" and "were" are often confused, and this can truly irritate markers. The best remedy for these word confusions is a dictionary: a hard copy of a good dictionary or a reliable online dictionary will detail whether the word you are contemplating is a noun, adjective or verb and will advise correct spellings and meanings. Using a dictionary should not add too much time to your essay writing and will improve your mark inordinately. Alarmingly, many medical students seem to use the words "practice" and "practise" interchangeably. Although they may sound identical and look similar, they have very different meanings:

Practice is the noun (the part of speech referring to an object, concept, place or person).

Example: *The local GP Practice.* Here "Practice" refers to a place and is therefore a noun.

Example: *It is common practice to anaesthetise patients before an operation.* Here "practice" refers to a specific concept and code of conduct and is therefore a noun.

Practise is a verb (a word that describes an action or a "doing" word).

Example: *I practised my note making.* Here "practised" refers to a specific action and so is a verb.

Example: *I realised that I will need to practise this skill more in the future.* Here "practise" refers to an action and is therefore a verb.

An easy way to remember the difference between practICE and practISE is that "ice" is a cold thing (a noun) and "ise" is not a thing. Another similar confusion is *"advice"* and *"advise"*. Fortunately those words follow the same rule.

USING ABBREVIATIONS

Certain abbreviations including "e.g.", "i.e." and "etc." are not appropriate in academic writing. Preferable alternatives could be "for example" or "that is" or "and so forth". It is, however, permissible to use abbreviations for medical terms after you have mentioned them in full once.

REFLECTING ON YOUR REFLECTIVE ESSAY

Once your essay has been marked and returned, another phase of reflection must ensue where you carefully read any annotations, comments or advice your tutor has made. As well as celebrating positive feedback, it is also vital that you carefully consider the targets you have been set to determine how you can prevent similar mistakes from impeding your work in the future. Thorough reflection is worthwhile: it will allow you to identify target areas and consider how to strengthen your own performance and progress. Reflection is key to improvement and achievement.

CHAPTER 3

The essays

Since commencing clinics, clerking and conversing with patients has played a major part in my education. Every experience with a patient has been very different and there have been a few times when taking the history has been less than easy. One clerking where this has been apparent involved two of my peers and I. This was the only time when I have clerked with two others and this was due to the clerking being a part of a future presentation.

One of the main problems in taking the history was the fact that the structure in which the clerking was taken was not the way I would have adopted if clerking alone. When trying to direct the clerking in a certain direction, this was reversed by a question by another student. As a result the length of the clerking was very long. The clerking with respect to this was very frustrating for me. Initially I repeatedly attempted to steer the clerking to the structure I work with best but after a few minutes I felt liked stopping asking the patient questions and letting the other two continue. I felt that we were not attaining the information we needed and thought as a result the clerking would not be sufficient to present. Therefore I also reduced my note taking, knowing that the person who was leading the clerking now was taking extensive notes. My mind-set was to give up with the clerking and go and find another patient. As a result I was not listening intently to what the patient was saying and possibly more significantly was not noticing how the patient was feeling.

When looking back at the situation, my thoughts and behaviors were very unprofessional in some sense. It would have been good to stay supportive to my team and help them more with questioning. However I feel that possibly by standing back from the clerking allowed the other two students to pursue their structure of clerking more effectively. However this was not going through my mind at the time.

Analysing the situation more intensely, the whole incident seems to show that I should possibly be more tolerant of others. This seems essential in order to work cohesively in a team. It also seems to show that I like certain things done in a specific way and possibly I should be more open to alternative ideas. However in another sense, after talking to the other two students after the clerking, we all felt as if it had not gone well due to the lack of structure of our questions collectively. Therefore the real obstacle may have been that we did not have a strategy discussed before talking to the patient, in order to make the clerking more efficient.

This clerking differs considerably to other clerkings which I have done. Usually either myself or one other student clerks a patient. With just one other person I have not been frustrated before because it has been more of a team effort, where if one person is struggling for questions, the other can come in to take the lead. With three however, everybody was trying to get their questions across, almost battling with the others to take control. Overlooking the event, if this situation were to present itself again and two students and I had to clerk a patient, I would suggest that each of us should tackle a certain section of the clerking by ourselves. This would allow for each person's strategy of clerking to not be disturbed. This would likely result in the clerking to flow more easily and be more time-efficient. However ideally, I would not recommend having three people clerk a patient again

COMMENTS ON REFLECTION

This is an interesting incident on which to reflect; a situation where, on further rumination, the author is able to identify that the incident has highlighted a flaw in his behaviour that he can see has the potential to cause problems in his professional work. The author has also reflected that his "in the moment" actions were wrong. This recognition and insight is momentous and illustrates the power and purpose of reflective practice. The student does not share with us his further thoughts about what he will learn from this experience, and this is a deficiency in the essay that leaves it incomplete. We do not know how this obviously mindful and insightful individual might go about dealing with this issue or the associated difficulties he anticipates.

The last two paragraphs are a disappointment to the reader. Instead of pressing on with this reflection he backtracks, expressing other, more favourable versions of his actions, which the reader might doubt.

COMMENTS ON ENGLISH

What was done well

➤ This piece of work is sensibly organised into logical paragraphs that reflect shifts in time, action and thought. Investing some time and thought into organising your essay into such paragraphs is worthwhile and your reader will be grateful to you for your planning.

What could have been done better

➤ This essay contains many unclear and long-winded sentences that are incredibly confusing to follow; the essay would have been much improved by keeping the sentences and structure simple and concise. The following example is far too complicated and needs to be read at least twice. A reader should be able to read and understand your writing with ease and enjoyment, so make sure that your sentences are completely clear, logical and understandable. Get into the habit of insisting each sentence says what you want it to say, simply and concisely. Don't make your readers work hard to understand what you want to tell them.

Original student version

When trying to direct the clerking in a certain direction, this was reversed by a question by another student. As a result the length of the clerking was very long. The clerking with respect to this was very frustrating for me.

Amended version

While I was taking the history, my fellow student's questions diverted the patient from my line of questioning, slowing down the history taking, and I found this frustrating.

➤ This essay also suffers from tense confusion. As reflective writing deals with an incident that took place in the past, which you then consider in present and future terms, a range of tenses are often used. However, you must have a firm and consistent grasp of the tenses in your writing, otherwise the chronology is confusing and the narrative is clumsy.

Original student version

When looking back at the situation, my thoughts and behaviours were very unprofessional in some sense. It would have been good to stay supportive to my team and help them more with questioning. However I feel that possibly by standing back from the clerking allowed the other two students to pursue their structure of clerking more effectively.

Amended version

When looking back at the situation, I realise that my thoughts and behaviour were very unprofessional. I should have been more supportive to my team and should have helped them with their questions. By not interrupting their history taking I probably allowed them to take the history more effectively.

Description: During one night shift on MAAU, an FY2 doctors asked for my immediate help. We went to the bedside of an 84 year old man who had been admitted due to CAP, and was a nursing home resident.

It was immediately apparent he was critically ill - his skin was waxy white and mottled. The FY2 was attempting to insert a femoral line, as no other veins were accessible, for a final fluid challenge.

My role was to restrain him by holding his arms and his legs, as he was very confused – his GCS was 9 – and visibly distressed. He was blind in both eyes and partially deaf. As I held him down, I tried to comfort him and explain what was happening. He repeatedly stroked my hands and mumbled someone's name.

It took 5 attempts for the line to be inserted. Towards the end, a nurse restrained him while I assisted the FY2. Once the line was inserted a registrar came to suction mucus from his airways. Again I was asked to restrain him. Both the registrar and I were shocked to see dark blood and reasoned that the man had either aspirated a GIT bleed or had a pulmonary haemorrhage.

After this I had to leave to attend a ward round. On returning later the man had died.

Emotions: Initially I was extremely shocked by the man's appearance. Despite having seen many cadavers and ill patients, I had never seen someone this critically ill or such widespread mottling. I was surprised by the doctor's response as she was furious that she had not been bleeped earlier when she might have been able to help this man effectively. I also felt uncomfortable with my role of 'restrainer'; one reason why I want to be a doctor is to try and minimise pain, and while I understand this sometimes involves transient pain, this case felt helpless and I wasn't convinced that my infliction of pain would ever be to his benefit. Finally I was unsure of the ethics of the situation as this man was certainly incapable of giving consent and I wasn't sure that the procedure was in his best interests. My feelings were shared by the registrar and also by the FY2 although she felt that this should be tried as a last attempt.

Outcomes: Ultimately the patient died but by comforting him as I did I was able to support him emotionally. The FY2 felt as if she had done everything in her power to prevent this man's death. The registrar, although admitting that he would not have tried to initiate a fluid challenge, understood the reasons why the FY2 had decided to do so. I learnt a little about the management of a critically ill patient and also saw the compassionate side of doctors, which isn't always overtly displayed. However, another consequence for me was concern about whether I had done the right thing to restrain a man seemingly against his will for a procedure I was unsure was in his best interests.

Evaluations: I was helping keep this man alive long enough to receive further treatment for his CAP. This was a philanthropic action which I felt uncomfortable with; was it appropriate if the degree of ischaemic damage already incurred meant that his future quality of life could be seriously impinged upon, and when his previous quality of life in a nursing home was not optimal?

Analysis: I was influenced by the immediate response to commands from a superior and the wish to do everything possible to maintain life. I was also influenced by my pursuit of knowledge to learn about femoral lines insertion. Finally I was influenced by the enjoyment of being part of a team, as so often medical students are observers rather than integral players.

The knowledge that this man would die without my help certainly influenced me but ethically it worried me. My difficulty lay in whether this was the best for the patient or whether offering more palliative treatment would have been appropriate, and so whether my behaviour was conflicting with my convictions.

Conclusions: Looking back on the experience I still feel upset by it, but predominantly by the fact that the situation arose at all e.g. why wasn't the patient in ITU? Why wasn't he being frequently monitored by the nursing staff, and why wasn't the doctor called to intervene at a much earlier stage? Whilst at the time I wasn't sure if it was in the patient's best interests, I am now glad that we did try as he warranted an attempted resuscitation. I think I acted as well as I could - I kept calm and was essential in my job of keeping the patient peaceful. I am also grateful that I could help someone during a frightening experience and make him believe he was being cared for by someone dear to him.

This was the first time I have been faced with an ethical dilemma of this magnitude but I doubt that this will be the last time and so it is useful to have experienced it early in my medical career. Speaking to others doctors helped me to support myself as they comforted me and assured me I had acted appropriately. This will certainly help me to help others in future, as there is little education on dealing with death, despite it being the eventual cure to all diseases, and an expectation that doctors are immune to feelings of grief or guilt after the death of a patient.

In future, I would act the same way, as I believe I acted as best I could. It is difficult to merge the ethics that are taught in a stuffy lecture theatre with everyday situations on the wards and so this was a vital lesson in how crucial it is to have preformed principles at the front of the mind where they are easily accessible in an emergency.

COMMENTS ON REFLECTION

There is plenty of reflection here and the essay is good, illustrating the essence of reflective practice. It should not be assumed that all readers understand medical abbreviations, which should be avoided or explained. Subheadings help shape and structure the essay, but too many make a piece staccato and jolt the reader.

The author reached an early conclusion that a vigorous attempt to resuscitate a very unwell patient was inappropriate, unlikely to succeed and, therefore, ethically questionable. This is a mature conclusion from an undergraduate. The author has described the clinical state of the patient appropriately, she has described her discomfort at being asked to restrain the patient during the protracted femoral vein cannulation and the pain she believed she inflicted, and the ethics of the attempt. How would the author have felt had the cannulation been successful after only one attempt and the resuscitation successful? Would she still have considered it "unethical" to try? Were her initial thoughts and emotions shaped by the outcome rather than the intention to treat, or simply inexperience? Interestingly, in her conclusion, and after reflection, she thought that intervention was appropriate. This is a very important statement highlighting her intellectual and emotional journey during the case. She probably would have come to the same conclusions had she not performed this formal written reflection but she may have forgotten it. It is possible that this reflective essay including her evaluation, analysis and conclusion will provide her with a major learning experience. This is the purpose of reflective writing.

COMMENTS ON ENGLISH
What was done well
➤ This essay is generally written in a clear and sophisticated way. Whilst ambitious vocabulary is used to aid precision of expression, the sentences are not overloaded with pompous-sounding and inappropriate words. The "Emotions" section here is particularly strong for these reasons. Words seem to have been carefully and thoughtfully selected but the sentences are straightforward and simple to follow.

What could have been done better
➤ The student has divided her work with sensibly named subtitles but the paragraph breaks are less admirable. This essay is littered with unfinished-looking paragraphs, the shortest of which is just two sentences long. The "paragraph" in question could have easily been welded onto the previous paragraph, where it actually would have made a lot more sense. Remember that paragraph breaks are not arbitrary and random and should not break up every single event that you are recalling if that means that you have to change paragraph every three sentences.
➤ The first sentence ". . . an FY2 doctors . . ." is irritating and should have been picked up with proofreading. This should be done several times until you are completely happy with your work.

As I have progressed through the medicine course, I have spoken to many patients and encountered various medical conditions, learning the pathological mechanisms behind them, how they can be treated and also the most common symptoms patients present with. The more patients I meet, the more often I notice that the severity of symptoms can appear much greater in an anxious or depressed patient.

The first time I truly encountered this issue was in the Accident and Emergency department one night. A 54 year old lady, Mrs K, came in complaining of two weeks of chest pain and shortness of breath. As we spoke to her, I got the overall impression of a very anxious woman, who probably felt rather lost and depressed after her husband's sudden death and felt particularly helpless since her son's serious accident, because he was in Cyprus and she was not able to be with him. I could imagine that she was quite lonely, with some of her children in Cyprus, and only the younger, teenaged children with her in England. She was very anxious throughout our conversation, explaining her many medical problems, and worrying about being a burden on her teenage daughter, who had to help her with most daily activities, including dressing. After a while, the doctor came to speak to the patient, and spent some time listening to Mrs K's concerns and quietly reassuring her that the tests showed no significant problems and that she could go home. As she was leaving the hospital, Mrs K seemed much less distressed and said she felt better.

I came across a similar situation when an elderly lady came to see the doctor in an outpatients clinic because of a fall she had had due to sudden dizziness. She walked in with the help of her walking stick, but seemed quite stable on her feet and looked well. However, she wore sunglasses throughout the consultation, sat hunched forward and spoke very quietly. It had been established that her dizzy spells were due to bradycardia, and the doctor had to explain to her that the pauses in her heartbeat were not long enough for a pacemaker to be of much use in preventing her dizziness. At this point the patient became very upset because she was so afraid of falling again. It emerged that she was a very lonely woman, with no family and few friends, and I imagine that she felt that there was no one to help her if she had another fall. I was very impressed by the way the doctor talked to the patient. She sat closer to her, held her hand and spoke very soothingly. She explained the situation in many different ways until she managed to convince the patient that she does not need a pacemaker. She also listened attentively and acknowledged her anxiety about falling. The patient began to cry and it seemed that she simply needed someone to talk to about her problems and fears. By the end of the consultation it was obvious that the doctor had won the patient's trust, and the patient walked out of the room with much more confidence than when she had come in.

Another time I saw the same issue was in a GP surgery. An 83 year old Turkish lady, Mrs I, came in with her daughter, who translated for her. We discovered that Mrs I had suffered from diabetes for many years, but insisted on having sweet snacks between meals. Her daughter believed that a high glucose level causes the tiredness, which prevents Mrs I from walking more than a few steps in the flat. It seemed Mrs I's daughter was usually her only contact, since she spent every day with her mother, from morning until evening, and brought her to stay with her family during weekends. We asked if Mrs I's symptoms change with her mood, and her daughter confirmed that even the weather can affect their severity. After examining the patient, the doctor suggested to try to improve the glucose control, but also recommended that Mrs I's daughter should get in touch with some sort of Turkish group in the community so that Mrs I could have more social contact. Although Mrs I could not understand what the doctor had advised, since her daughter had not translated it yet, after the consultation she seemed happier and I believe she responded to the doctor's calm speech and the general impression that he understands and acknowledges her problems.

Seeing these three women made me realise how big an influence a patient's mood has on symptoms. Loneliness and depression may cause a patient to focus more on their own symptoms and seek medical attention because they are afraid, have no one to turn to for reassurance, and feel it is out of their control. Anxiety may exaggerate the seriousness of the situation in the patient's eyes and they may simply need to be listened to and assured that someone will take care of them. The three patients, in whom the effects of anxiety and depression particularly struck me, all came to see a doctor worried that they have a serious medical problem. All three women walked away from their doctor with much more confidence, their symptoms no longer seeming so serious and frightening. Although in the medical course so far I have been trying to learn how to treat various medical conditions, these three cases in particular made me realise that sometimes, when no significant treatment is needed, it is equally important to simply take time to listen to the patient, ask them about their social situation, try to understand what is causing their anxiety, and if possible comfort them and assure them that it is not out of control. I have also observed consultations after which patients walk away obviously unfulfilled, and I have realised how much of a difference it makes to recognise a patient's worries, reassure them and see them leave feeling much more optimistic.

COMMENTS ON REFLECTION

There is very little personal reflection in this essay. It is almost entirely descriptive. We do not know how the author felt about each encounter, whether she felt anything could have been done better or how she might have behaved if she had been responsible for the care of each patient. Whilst listening carefully to patients, analysing what is wrong, excluding other serious conditions and giving reassurance is an important part of medicine, it appears that the author already knew this and so has not learned anything new from these experiences.

For a reflective essay, it is usually more sensible to concentrate on one case, describe briefly the clinical circumstances, and then reflect. Here, the reader is given descriptions of three separate events and then a summary sentence. If the author had reflected on only one episode, explored how she felt about the patient and doctor interaction, the motivations and actions of the two parties, whether there might have been different approaches, whether this might have created different outcomes and how she might have approached things differently, it is likely that she would have learned more and written a more cogent and interesting essay.

COMMENTS ON ENGLISH

What was done well

➤ This essay is logically ordered and well paragraphed. The reader can easily track events and the scenarios described because the narrative moves and develops in a sensible way. Despite various spelling and grammatical errors, the introduction here is particularly effective as it is prepares the reader for the reflection.

What could have been done better

➤ There are a few areas of careless spelling, typing and grammar. Whilst the opening paragraph is thematically good, it is grammatically poor. Opening and closing paragraphs are often the most memorable, whether that be for good or bad reasons, and it is regrettable that the introduction is littered with bad typing and grammar. The second sentence is also strangely ordered and requires a few rereadings. Your sentences should always make sense first time round and, unless you are a very confident and accomplished writer, you should usually stick to simple phrasing to make it easy for your reader.

Original student version

As I have progressed through the medicine course, I have spoke to many patients and encountered various medical conditions, learning the pathological mechanisms behind them, how they can be treated and also the most common symptoms patients present with. The more patients I meet, the more often I notice that the severity of symptoms can appear much greater in an anxious or depressed patient.

Amended version

During my clinical course, I have clerked many patients with various medical conditions, and learned about the underlying pathology and treatments. I have also learned about common symptoms and have been struck with the way that symptoms reflect a patient's mood and emotions; symptoms are often worse in anxious and depressed patients, compared with patients who are calm and optimistic.

➤ The essay has some awkward sentences that are usually too long and badly constructed. Again, this detracts from the overall impression of the work. You can improve the fluidity of your work by proofreading it; breaking long sentences down into shorter ones and adding connective words or phrases to improve coherence and ensuring that all tenses agree with one another.

Original student version

Although Mrs I could not understand what the doctor had advised, since her daughter had not translated it yet, after the consultation she seemed happier and I believe she responded to the doctor's calm speech and the general impression that he understands and acknowledges her problems.

Amended version

Although Mrs I could not understand what the doctor had advised, since her daughter had not translated it yet, she seemed happier after the consultation. I believe she responded well to the doctor's calm speech, which gave her the impression that he understood and acknowledged her problems.

This was the first time on a ward round that I had felt uncomfortable. In front of me was a nervous 80 year old lady and on my right was the registrar conducting the ward round. The confrontation was very calm, quiet and controlled but disquieting at the same time. They were discussing what should happen next in the patient's care. She wanted to go home because she had lots of things to do. The registrar on the other hand was insistent that she stay to undergo further tests.

The patient would not be persuaded to stay in hospital for longer. She was very polite but visibly perturbed by the doctor's behaviour and worried by what might happen to her if she left the hospital. She didn't want to stay in the hospital because she could not be guaranteed the tests would be carried out quickly. She didn't divulge why she had to rush home which I found difficult to comprehend. At that time, I found it difficult to understand her position but this was overridden by the registrar's behaviour.

The registrar was smiling away, but obviously offended that the patient would not acquiesce to his demands and tried repeatedly to convince her to follow his plan rather than respecting her opinions. His approach was overbearing and attempted scare tactics to encourage her to change her mind. Moreover, he was using medical jargon which was both confusing and frightening the patient. At no point did he stop to explain what the tests were or why they had to be done. I think he knew that his tests were important but not essential to the patient who was stable and asymptomatic. It was quite frustrating to hear the conversation take place because the patient was distressed and the doctor could have taken more time and care to explain both his case and what he proposed.

Whilst this was occurring, I and the other two students stood on the other side to the patient and registrar observing the consultation. I didn't speak up because I didn't fully know the situation, and felt the doctor was in a better position to judge. Not only that, but I thought it was better to be respectful to the registrar who let us follow him on the ward round rather than contradict him. This was in spite of the patient's plaintive looks for support and relief from us students. The FY1 was busy writing in the notes and trying to avoid the gaze of the patient.

Eventually, the registrar relented and a compromise was reached. The patient would go home that day, but would come back in at a later date for the tests. This was obviously not the optimum result from his point of view, but the only one the patient was ready to accept. I was shocked at how long he had persisted trying to win round the patient and disregarding their opinion for so long. He seemed so intent on imposing his will that he couldn't accept any other viewpoint.

My first reaction was that he was ignoring her wishes with the best intentions – trying to protect the patient and making the care of the patient his first priority. However, I couldn't justify his actions to others and am still unable to. Plus, it appeared as if he wasn't treating the patient as an individual and respecting her decision, more as someone who was incapable of making the right decision. This was exacerbated by not explaining the tests to her. To me, this highlighted the superiority of the doctor and the faith he placed in his opinion over his respect for the patient's right to reach decisions on their own. Ultimately, he conceded and tried to work with the patient and listened to what she preferred, but this was delayed by his actions. My second reaction was to say something to the doctor and try to dissuade him from carrying on. I didn't interrupt at all. We left the patient without trying to reassure her that her decision was valuable too, and worried. I agreed with the doctor that the tests needed to be done, but not at the expense of the patient's state of mind.

I felt that she wanted some respite and supportive words that she would be ok to leave the hospital. I think this moment stood out because with a patient centred view of medicine, the patients beliefs and ideas are as important as the doctors. Despite this, I was left squirming at the side believing that my opinion was not as important as the two people in front of me. I think if I had the opportunity again, I would not have stepped in because I still believe that I was not fully informed on the situation. Instead I would have tried to return later on in the day and possibly try to find out why she was so keen to leave and troubling her at home. Even if I would not be able to convince her from a clinical perspective, I might have been able to comfort her on a personal level.

On that day, I could have attempted to make an impact on that patient's care, assuming she wanted to have another stranger to speak to, but I didn't. It was probably a combination of inexperience and lack of confidence which stopped me from attempting it. I think I have learnt to listen to the patient's opinions rather than impose my medical knowledge and training.

If this situation occurred again, I hope that I would trust myself and tried to offer the patient some respite, or at the very least go back and speak to her.

COMMENTS ON REFLECTION

This essay starts out well, with two brief descriptive paragraphs setting the scene and describing the author's discomfort with the registrar's attempt to keep the patient in hospital for further tests against her will. The reader feels this is going to develop into a good reflective analysis but, instead, the author continues on with more and more description. We are told that, after much negotiation and discussion, the patient "won" her right to be discharged and to be investigated as an outpatient. There are many unaddressed issues in this essay. The author relates that the registrar used medical jargon. What jargon was used? How did he know that the patient did not understand this? How would the author have conducted the consultation and how would he have dealt with the patient? Was there any justification for the registrar's insistence that the patient should stay in to complete the tests? Did the author think that the registrar's stance was inappropriate and, if so, how did he feel about this? Did the author have sympathy for the registrar? By the sixth paragraph we get some reflection-on-action but it is superficial. Why might the registrar be acting in this way? Why did the author feel at the time that he could not intervene? Why does he not feel the same way now? What makes him think he would act differently next time?

The patient wanted to go home and, like any other patient, she had the right to refuse treatment and tests. Patients do not have to have a reason for non-consent. Doctors are only advisors but have to give patients sufficient understandable factual information so that patients can make their own adequately informed decision. The author does not reflect on this but restricts his essay to the registrar's manner during the consultation.

The author describes himself as a "stranger" but he wasn't and isn't: he was an integral part of this scene. Had he recognised this role, he may perhaps have written a better reflective piece rather than devote such a large proportion of the piece to description.

COMMENTS ON ENGLISH
What was done well

➤ This essay is generally well paragraphed. Although the last sentence is isolated and is definitely not of the length or topical independence to warrant such separation, the rest of the essay is logically ordered and divided into paragraphs to reflect the development of situation and thought process.

What could have been done better

➤ The general quality of the English in this work is not bad at all but it is clear that the student did not proofread the essay carefully before submission because there are a number of various grammatical mistakes that should have been corrected. Inadequate proofreading is a common fault in the reflective essays we see and this is regrettable and unnecessary. The first example of inadequate proofreading shows that some pronouns have been omitted, leaving the reader confused about who was trying to convince whom. The improved version clarifies the subject and object, the sentence has been split into two to make it easier to read, and both sentences should now make sense to the reader. Short sentences are usually easier to read and understand than long ones.

Original student version
The registrar was smiling away, but obviously offended that the patient would not acquiesce to his demands and tried repeatedly to convince her to follow his plan rather than respecting her opinions.

Amended version
The registrar was smiling but he was obviously offended that the patient would not agree to stay in hospital. Rather than respecting her opinions, he tried repeatedly to convince her to follow his plan.

➤ Another awkward phrase reads: "I and the other two students stood on the other side". If the student had read this aloud they probably would have realised that, although it is grammatically correct, it sounds awkward. A better, more fluid alternative could be: "I stood with the two other students on the other side". Proofreading your essay at least twice is essential.

➤ Many medical students confuse tenses when writing reflectively. The nature of reflective writing, pausing to look back on a situation to aid current progress and future practice, demands a firm and stable grasp of the past, present, future and conditional tenses: *I did that, I do that, I will do that, I would do that*. This extract shows tense confusion and inappropriate use of the word "respite". Remember, keep your sentences clear, concise and simple.

Original student version
If this situation occurred again, I hope that I would trust myself and tried to offer the patient some respite, or at the very least go back and speak to her.

Amended version
If this situation occurred again, I would go back to speak to the patient to explain why I thought she should stay in hospital.

Description and Outcomes of Event

In a recent Orthopaedic outpatient clinic I was asked by my Registrar to take a history and examine a patient in front of him. Mrs CS was a 59 year old attending for a check up relating to her diagnosis of osteoarthritis. When Mrs CS entered the consulting room it was instantly apparent that she was morbidly obese.

Mrs CS's size raised a number of issues. I began by taking a history, but was wary of unduly offending by questioning her about her weight. However, I endeavoured not to make assumptions so routinely asking a thorough social history including an assessment of her diet, exercise and ADLs. Her presenting complaint was of bilateral knee pain, worsened by movement.

On examining the knee joint it is necessary to assess the patient's passive movement putting the legs into full flexion; this meant that I was taking the whole weight of her leg. On the one hand this risked damaging me musculoskeletally by lifting such a weight. On the other hand I could have damaged the patient by moving her incorrectly. Another problem on examination was palpating the joint margins; with such a degree of subcutaneous fat this was virtually impossible, thus reducing the sensitivity of the examination.

In terms of treatment I observed the doctor injecting steroid and local anaesthetic into the knee joints. I asked the doctor how he could locate the joint when we had been unable to palpate any joint lines. He replied that it was basically guesswork and he'd just go down until he hit bone then come up again. This method is not accurate, may cause the patient pain on execution and may elucidate no lasting benefit.

Emotions

Reflecting on the episode, I admit that my initial feeling was one of revulsion. Mrs CS's legs were ripples of fat, bulging out of her shoes. When I came to examine her the growth of fungal infection between these roles emitted an unpleasant smell.

I was also exasperated because it became clear from earlier correspondence that Mrs CS had been advised to lose weight in order to prevent her osteoarthritis getting any worse.

The doctor said that Mrs CS would still be a candidate for a Total Knee Replacement(TKR) if steroid injections did not help, regardless of the fact that her weight could make the operation risky and she might gain little from it if she continued to remain inactive. I found this surprising, and in my head questioned the benefit to Mrs CS and the sense in allocation of NHS resources.

I did however, I hope, maintain a polite friendly outward demeanour throughout the consultation.

Evaluation

The positive side to this encounter was that both I and the doctor performed to an expected level in terms of thorough history taking and examination. Although the latter was difficult, the doctor who carried out the steroid injection was experienced enough to be fairly certain of a positive result. In terms of follow up support and appointments, there was still a clear opportunity for the patient to have the necessary TKR if needed and I believe the patient left the consultation feeling satisfied with events. Personally, it was my first encounter with such a morbidly obese patient, and it forced me to go away and reflect on the consultation, my reaction and associated issues of accountability for obesity, allocation of NHS resources and doctor attitudes to obesity.

On a negative note, the patient's size meant that the examination was not as good as it should have been. I question whether the treatment will prove as effective as it has the potential to be. In terms of reaction, I was ashamed by my own revulsion, and saddened by the doctor's flippancy with regard to patient pain and inefficacy of treatment.

Analysis

It is easy to polarise views on obesity, for example:

1. The patient is wholly to blame for being "lazy"; they should eat less and exercise more. Patients who are morbidly obese should be denied treatments such as TKR because they have brought osteoarthritis on themselves and thus do not deserve it. They would not benefit from the operation and would use up resources that a slimmer person could better use.
2. Obesity is 80% genetic and thus the patient's lifestyle is not to blame. They might want to exercise to lose weight but their pre-existing osteoarthritis makes movement too painful. By giving them a TKR it could not only improve pain, but allow exercise and thus improve symptoms associated with obesity as well as increasing quality of life. This would also reduce the pressure on the NHS by reducing morbidity.

In the case of Mrs CS, I do not think patient care was actually compromised by the play of these paradoxical views. However, what the situation did highlight to me was the complex nature of the issue of obesity for medical professionals. Obesity cannot simply be polarised in terms of causality or attitudes to its effect on treatment from the doctor's point of view. Actions and events associated with obesity may be "located within and explicable by multiple perspectives, but are located in and influenced by multiple and socio-political contexts." The doctor may be influenced by past experiences of overweight people, by studies about its effect on morbidity, their own personal experiences of weight, their beliefs about perceived causality of a patient's obesity and their beliefs about priorities in the NHS. This may be detrimental to patient care. What is more, it seems more and more patients are unwilling to seek help from doctors because of the public perception that doctors judge their overweight patients.

From a personal point of view there were a number of factors influencing me: my gut reaction, my training to present a polite professional manner, my desire to impress the Registrar, my wish to have a rapport with both the doctor and the patient. With my knowledge of what is required of a medical student, and my personal values on how people should be treated, I subconsciously made the decision to elicit an examination to the best of my ability, and to treat the patient well. Nonetheless, I am still ashamed of some of my derisive attitudes to obesity, which may well be born of lack of education. Thus there was a degree of incongruity between how I would consciously wish to act, and how I felt.

Conclusions

In general, I would conclude that as physicians it is necessary to think about our attitudes to obesity and how this on the one hand affects our handling of patients, and on the other hand affects how the medical profession is perceived.

As a medical student this was my first clinical experience of examining an obese patient. Having reflected on some of the issues surrounding obesity and its perception, I now think that I would handle future patients with more respect mentally, and endeavour to maintain a good level of patient care. In the future I would not be as daunted by the prospect of eliciting a successful examination of an obese patient, and I think I would be less quick to judge.

BBC, 'Fat equals lazy , say doctors', http://news.bbc.co.uk/1/hi/health/3143012.stm, last updated 27/09/03, [accessed 14/11/09]

BBC, 'Obese bias' concern for patients, http://news.bbc.co.uk/1/hi/scotland/8070989.stm, last updated 27/05/09, [accessed 14/11/09]

COMMENTS ON REFLECTION

This is a well-structured reflective piece. It is written honestly, analytically, personally and with insight. The author felt uncomfortable with the way she felt about this patient and confessed that her feelings were unprofessional, unfair and due to lack of clinical experience.

Obesity is a complex condition with major medical complications, and financial implications for the NHS and health services. Medical students may feel uncomfortable writing about obesity because they feel it upsets or "offends" the patient by making personal comments about their appearance, so this is a brave choice.

Is the author's guilt about feeling repulsed by the patient's obesity inappropriate or wrong? Health workers should not let their personal views influence any aspect of their professional approach or clinical management decision. Students and doctors are human and have human reactions to illnesses. Revulsion in these circumstances is a good subject for reflection: what impact does such a powerful emotion have on a consultation? What can one do to mitigate the effects of these powerful emotions? The author's guilt is misplaced. It could be argued that doctors who do not and cannot speak or write honestly about their emotions are incomplete doctors. This is of course one of the reasons for reflective practice.

The author also claims to have felt "exasperated" with the patient's failure to comply with previous repeated advice about weight loss. This, again, is a good reaction to reflect on but what, exactly, is making the author exasperated? Is it simply frustration with the patient's non-compliance? It would have been interesting to learn the cause of her feelings.

This author in this essay has used references. Unless your course encourages this,

these are not necessary in a piece that is about the author rather than the area of medical practice.

COMMENTS ON ENGLISH
What was done well
➤ This essay is well planned and structured. The sequence of events and associated thought process is clear and, although the subheadings are not totally necessary, the reader has no problem tracking the developments described in this essay.
➤ Vocabulary is carefully chosen to convey precise emotions. Words such as "daunted", "derisive" and "elucidate" are not only ambitious but also interesting to read. Varying vocabulary makes writing exciting to read and to write and it is worthwhile investing in a thesaurus or using an electronic one to source interesting words. However, you must take care when selecting words from a thesaurus to ensure they are appropriate and loyal to your meaning, and if English is not your first language it is worth asking a colleague or friend who does speak English as a first language to make sure that your choice of words is appropriate and correct.

What could have been done better
➤ Whilst some of the paragraphs are well formed and ordered, others are disconcertingly short and comprised of isolated sentences. Whilst you may spot sentence-long paragraphs in newspapers, they are rarely appropriate in academic work as they seem undeveloped and rushed. The "Emotions" section of the essay is full of isolated sentences that could be easily and seamlessly fitted onto the preceding paragraphs. In general, a paragraph should be at least three sentences long.

I was on my critical care placement conducting a DRABCDE algorithm on a patient who had been admitted with a perforated gall bladder. The gentleman we were to be examining was clearly ill, but not to a critical degree and was clearly competent and able to even issue a few quips during the process of investigation. It was not him that we were worried about.

It was his wife that was to be the crux of the issue and is now the focus of my piece. From her diminutive frame, sat beside her husband, she darted venomous looks and her general complexion was that of a lady scorned; she clearly did not want us to be there. This was in stark juxtaposition to her husband's friendly demeanour and charm, despite the presence of a venture mask strapped around his face. With every letter of the algorithm reached her face grew sourer and we became faster in our consultation, to the extent that I measured capillary refill time having squeezed the patient's finger for less than a second, a less than satisfactory testing time. I felt quite intimidated by her presence and slightly agitated; I wanted to leave as soon as possible.

We hastily completed our analysis, thanked the patients and relatives present and made for the corridor as quickly as possible. Upon regrouping, our clinical tutor explained that he had no problems consenting the patient for the brief exercise but the wife had been challenge. As we reflected on our discoveries, working through the DRABCDE algorithm, we all agreed that the Danger section should include relatives, for the wife's presence had dramatically affected our consultation. With the notes documented and the session over I began to reflect (and am still reflecting as I type now) as to way I had conducted myself during that investigation.

Clearly DRABCDE is of the utmost importance for medical students to be familiar with. As a FY1 doctor I am sure this algorithm will aid me in dealing with what can be very distressing and high pressure situations, its magnitude is of no doubt. Teaching it on dummies in a clinical skills lab however, is very different to the real thing. There are many factors that come into play on the wards and the presence of relatives is a major one. Had the wife not had been there then the entire process of DRABCDE would have been completed more thoroughly at a leisurely pace perhaps more conducive to learning. However, it is easy for one to forget how protective family are. Families obviously are defensive of their own and the thought of snotty nosed medical students poking about their ill loved ones makes this impulse to shield them even stronger. It is an entirely understandable response, yet it may seem unreasonable.

In this context the situation was confused by the consent of the patient being countered by the wrath of the wife. She was clearly devoted to her husband, and was willing to protect him from us, even at the cost of going against his word. As a doctor such a situation I imagine occurs often, perhaps not in such a duplicate fashion but more in terms of patient treatment. All treatments carry a risk, a risk the patient themselves is willing to take. Should the unfortunate happen and they cease to exist, it would be a passing onto another world or no world at all (depending on beliefs). Their light will extinguish, but their family members continue to burn bright alone or missing a key flame. And it is this fact that family members find most difficult to tackle emotionally. The thought of losing a loved one at times is greater than the personal fear of death; resulting in a hypersensitivity to risk associated with treatments of family members (or in this case an exercise involving medical students). Would I have done the same as the wife? As a medical student myself I would probably allow students, however, as a medical student I would be more acutely aware of risks and mistakes. Thus I imagine myself much like the wife, watching their actions like a hawk, making sure no one injured my beloved. As I mentioned earlier it is an understandable but mainly unreasonable response.

In the context of a medical student we are mostly powerless to intervene in such a situation. An obstinate relative is a tough challenge for a student whose remit covers little and experience is paltry. In this case even our clinical tutor admitted it was better to flee before being "chucked out". If the objection had been milder would I have attempted to negotiate? Probably, but one must be wary of causing distress to both relative and patient. The best one can do is to elaborate what is to be done to or with the patient as succinctly and clearly as possible so that both patient and relative can grasp the situation fully. Rarely as a medical student do you do anything terribly invasive, and of course one must stop if the patient is in any discomfort or pain.

Overall I would say what may on initial inspection seem to be a situation where you have a "silly angry wife" is actually upon   closer analysis an interesting ethical dilemma which raises a host of interesting questions. From this I have learned not to succumb to pressure from relatives when under their scrutiny, to not let them affect the quality of care I give to a patient and to my own learning. Upon reflection I have learnt to understand the situation from the relatives' perspective and see the importance of both the patient and the relative fully understanding what is going on. This whole process has hopefully made me a more confident student with a better grasp of the holistic treatment of patients and their families.

COMMENTS ON REFLECTION

This is a good subject for reflection and raises several complex issues, some of which the author touches on. This essay starts nicely and the reader is quickly brought into the incident. The description is relatively brief and, promisingly, the reader is told "I began to reflect (and am still reflecting as I type now) as to way I had conducted myself during that investigation". There is a lot of reflection; the author has explored his feelings about this experience, put himself in the position of the wife and has come to a firm conclusion about the importance of understanding how patients and their relatives feel about medical interventions. This is the whole point of reflective writing and the reader is persuaded that the author has, by opening his eyes to the emotions and views of all parties, learned a useful lesson. Most students could have come to similar conclusions, but only if they had the sense and sensibility to think in this way.

The rest of the piece is based on the assumption that the wife was aggressive towards the students because she did not want them to clerk her husband and the author feels that this is unreasonable behaviour: the "silly angry wife". This is an example of a student basing their reflection on an unexplored, superficial assumption and lack of understanding of the wife, her attitudes to her husband and his illness, and her mental state. Doctors and nurses often come to unfair, hasty conclusions about patients and their relatives and this can be very unhelpful to all parties.

We are given the impression by the choice of language throughout that the students and the clinical teacher have been wronged by an unpleasant and difficult woman. The phrase "a lady scorned" in this kind of piece is inappropriate. It seems that the students did not speak to the wife to explain what they were doing and did not obtain her consent. Had they done so, would this have got her "on side" without darting "venomous looks"?

We should not let our personal views about patients and what appears to be their "peculiarities" of character or lifestyle influence the way we treat them. First impressions can be totally wrong. Learning from these mistakes by "reflecting after action" is a useful way to help us learn, by seeing things more clearly. Using the phrase "Would I have done the same as the wife?" is a good way to do this by exploring another's perspective.

COMMENTS ON ENGLISH
What was done well

➤ The quality of the English here is very good. The work is structured well; the grammar is generally good; vocabulary choices are excellent and the sentences are well constructed and easy to follow. Sentence structure has been varied to make the reading experience interesting and the piece as a whole is very engaging.

What could have been done better

➤ There are no considerable issues or problems with the quality of the English in this essay.

The trust between a patient and doctor enables them to confide in doctors about intimate issues that may be embarrassing. This essay discusses sexual problems in a man with bladder neck problems and my reflections about the consultation.

During my surgery firm, I was sitting in with a male urology registrar in a primarily female incontinence and bladder reconstruction clinic.

A married twenty-nine year old man of Islamic faith (Mr. SM) arrived at the urology clinic by himself for ongoing treatment for bladder neck sphincter dysnergia.

Mr. SM was informed by the registrar that I was a medical student and asked his permission if I could sit in on the consultation. He had no objection. Mr. SM had been given an alpha-blocker drug to relax the bladder neck to treat his symptoms. One side effect to this medication is retrograde ejaculation that presents with "whitish" urine, which the patient reported during this consultation. The registrar told me that it is much more common for the patient to experience normal, anterograde ejaculation rather than retrograde ejaculation.

Upon the registrar questioning the patient about this, Mr. SM did purposefully hesitate and look towards myself. The registrar noticed this and instantly insisted that I was indeed a medical student, informing the patient that I had scientific knowledge about masturbation, ejaculation, semen and sex and not to be embarrassed to talk of this in front of me. Mr. SM then continued talking but I sensed that he was still rather reluctant in doing so.

I was further surprised that the registrar himself did not re-offer the patient the option of whether I could stay or not at this point.

At this point, I thought that Mr. SM felt a little awkward and I had the instinct to offer to leave the consultation room, thinking that the patient had the right to ask me to leave if I did not offer myself. I was slightly shocked by the registrar's insinuations on how I should stay and so indirectly forcing the patient to talk about his retrograde ejaculation problem in front of me. I instantly wondered whether this was the right thing for the registrar to do.

In past clinics where this privacy issue has arisen, I have fully understood and obeyed instructions to leave after a patient's request for their privacy with the doctor. For example, when a doctor has to tell a patient that they have a terminal illness such as cancer, many students are asked to leave the room understandably for privacy. Again, we can only be taught in superficial scenarios of how to break such bad news but when it comes to seeing it done in practise by a professional, we are unable to do so even though it is for understandable reasons. Therefore I understand it can be difficult for students to see certain conditions and techniques for many reasons until perhaps in post-graduate training. This is where it can be problematic in finding a way around this and so I can understand why the registrar insisted on me staying without giving the patient a choice. As students, sitting in on clinics can be very helpful in observing communications techniques of a doctor as well as seeing different conditions and diseases which is why it is probably the best method of learning clinical medicine,

However, bearing in mind that the patient's best interest is of top priority, I wondered if this contraindicated the patient's privacy rights during a consultation?

After some thought, it did strike me to the dilemma of how medical students are supposed to learn and be exposed to conditions and communication techniques without infringing on patient's rights and choices in a clinical setting.

I wondered if Mr. SM was aware that he had the right to ask me to leave if he felt uncomfortable with my presence in this consultation. I assumed that he thought that he would be alone with the doctor and be able to talk more freely to him and so didn't anticipate a student to be there as well.

On my behalf, I thought I acted professionally, shy or not of hesitating to leave the room. I did not squirm or look away whilst Mr. SM was talking about his problems and did not react any differently as if he was telling us about simple toothache. I believe this helped him in feeling a little easier as if I looked down or showed my uneasiness in any way, Mr. SM may have sensed this and it would have only made it more difficult for him to talk honestly and openly about his problems to the registrar in front of me.

However, with the registrar also being of the same Asian ethnicity, his actions further surprised me. This was because I assumed that the registrar would have more greatly understood Mr. SM's reservations than anyone else and would have willing accounted for that.

I concluded that the experience of sitting in this consultation has bought to light something that had not greatly struck me before; the power a doctor has over a patient, even in overruling a patient's right, whether the patient is aware of this right or not, and despite whether it is beneficial or not to others like myself.

Also, as hard as it may be, not to make assumptions over patients and doctors as I could always be surprised and it could easily turn dangerous in other circumstances.

Even though I doubted whether Mr. KR did the right thing of not giving Mr. SM the choice of whether I could stay or not, I can understand and appreciate the reasons he did this. I am also proud of the way I acted professionally and indifferently to a sensitive and private topic for this patient and in a similar situation I would act no different.

COMMENTS ON REFLECTION

This piece is difficult to assess as a piece of reflective writing. The first half does not focus on the issue in hand and throughout the whole piece it alternates among breaking bad news, the over-forceful registrar, the author's own feelings of wanting to leave and the patient's feelings. The author never quite pins down or explains what is troubling him. The reader is left wondering what the author is reflecting on and what he has learned.

The paragraph that starts "I concluded that the experience . . ." is the most important part of the piece with regard to the potential for thinking about personal growth. This discussion, unfortunately, then fizzles out. The author needs to move on to explore what this experience means for future practice and how he can avoid abusing power, purposefully or unintentionally.

COMMENTS ON ENGLISH
What was done well

➤ The opening two sentences of this essay are excellent. A clear, concise and relevant introduction is integral to reflective writing. Introductions should succinctly explain what you are reflecting on and the significance of the incident to you on a personal and professional level. Although the introduction here is not perfectly worded, it defines the parameters of the essay quite effectively.

What could have been done better

➤ This essay is badly paragraphed. A paragraph break should indicate a slight shift in topic or time and should constitute at least three sentences to enable each paragraph and thought to develop effectively. Paragraphs that are too short can look like confusing suspended sentences. This essay contains numerous non-paragraphs that effectively make the thought process behind the essay seem slightly flighty and incoherent. The second and third paragraphs could be improved by simply linking them to each other and the fourth paragraph as they are all dealing with introducing the same incident in the same way.

➤ Parts of this essay are phrased in a rather unclear and clumsy way and require a few readings to make sense. Good written English is simple and should make sense on a first reading. Your tutor will become frustrated if they are forced to read and reread your work in order to make sense of it. Some of these sentences could have been improved by simplifying the grammar and reordering the sentences during the proofreading stages. If English is not your first language, perfecting word order and sentence construction (syntax) can be difficult. If you are unsure about your English, ask a competent peer to help you check your work.

➤ The following sentence contained a few grammatical glitches involving grammar and tense and needs to be refined and simplified:

Original student version

Upon the registrar questioning the patient about this, Mr. SM did purposefully hesitate and look towards myself.

Amended version

When the registrar questioned the patient about this, Mr SM purposefully hesitated and looked towards me.

While on MAAU, a patient was admitted with a paracetamol overdose. The patient was a quiet, soft-spoken and very pleasant man in his early fifties. He was a writer and readily acknowledged to having attempted suicide. He had a long history of mood disorders, mainly depression, but also anxiety, and possibly a manic episode in the past. He had, however, never previously attempted suicide.

A psychiatrist was called to assess his suicide risk and produce a judgement on how safe this patient was. This appears to be very good practice. Clearly, a psychiatrist would be the most well-placed specialist to pass such a judgement. As I have some nterest in psychiatry, I awaited the arrival of the psychiatrist eagerly, and was very nterested in seeing such an assessment first hand.

Before I proceed, I'd like to just make a couple of remarks about suicide. First, it kills about 1,000,000 people every year (Goldsmith et al., 2003; Mann et al., 2005). This is on the scale of mortality due to malaria. Are we, health professionals, any good at dealing with it? Maybe more specific to the present scenario, are we any good at assessing and predicting it? The evidence is scarce at best. Typing "suicide prediction" into Google Scholar or Pubmed yields but a handful of reviews. In a recent one, Oquendo et al. 2006 concluded that the only good predictors we have are of a past attempt and a refractory or recurrent depression. The problem, of course, is that these are not very specific predictors, and hence of limited clinical value. Other predictors have either not been replicated, or are in direct contradiction to each other. Prospective studies and studies aimed directly at the clinical setting have similarly revealed only little (Gaynes et al., 2004).

I was thus very excited to see how a liaison psychiatrist would deal with this conundrum. When he arrived, I joined him and met the patient. Unfortunately, the consultation was rather unsatisfactory. The psychiatrist had to leave three times to respond to a bleep. At least to me, there seemed to be very little structure in his discussion, and the history was certainly not thorough. In addition, I didn't feel like the immediate setting of the suicide attempt was explored in any significant way. When talking to the patient afterwards, he told me that the main stressor in his life was an elderly neighbour above him who made a lot of DIY noise, even at night. He said that this made it impossible for him to sleep—either the noise would wake him, or he would worry about the noise starting.

Of course, I have no idea of quite how accurate the assessment was. I also don't know if helping the patient with the stressor would have helped. Intuitively, it would seem that sending such a patient back to his home, where he is alone and reports significant distress might not be a good idea. But then, we just don't know. Certainly, had I attemped to commit suicide in my own home because I felt trapped here and exposed to the destructive whims of a neighbour, I would not want to just be sent back there after a weird night in a hospital. When I asked the patient directly, he said he would very much appreciate help with moving to a new flat, or somehow solving that situation. I suggested to him that he should mention this to the psychiatrist, and mentioned it to the psychiatrist myself.

I was struck very powerfully by a number of things. First, the situation. I wondered how I would react to it. Obviously, having just attempted suicide, I would be in a very complex mindset. Doctors have powerful impacts on patients. But I wonder what the effect of a psychiatrist would be on me in that situation. The psychiatrist told the patient a number of times that there were other ways out of this situation than suicide, and that he was of course interested in avoiding a suicide. Having just attempted suicide, I would probably have been struck by the superficiality of these statements. Of course, not committing suicide had been my goal throughout

a long period of suffering. I probably would have interpreted the psychiatrist's comments as not giving value to the suffering that led to the decision to take my life. Second, the rather shoddy assessment of a life-threatening condition. As pointed out above, suicide is a major cause of death across the world. The type of assessment that is brought to bear on it appears absolutely and miserably limited, compared to say the machinery that goes into action as soon as a breast cancer is suspected. Some of the unsatisfactory aspects of the assessment I witnessed were, I would argue, due to the psychiatrist. But to a large extent, the unpleasant aspects of the situation are simply due to the state at which psychiatry is. There simply are no good procedures to follow, there is no evidence advocating one approach over the other. It struck me that, at the end of the day, what disturbed me may well be utterly irrelevant in terms of outcomes for the patient.

Thus, and this was certainly the most distressing aspect to me personally, I was disappointed to see that the helplessness expressed in the literature on suicide finds such a drastic expression in daily clinical practice. It was very sad to see that, really, we had very little help to offer this gentle man.

During this event I was but an onlooker. I did attempt to interfere when I thought the situation at home had not been explored and addressed sufficiently. I am satisfied about the way in which I acted, given my knowledge. However, I do wish I had more understanding of the management of patients at risk of suicide. As a student, not even having done psychiatry, I do not feel like I had sufficient understanding to interfere any more. After all, I do not have good evidence to support that what I was suggesting would have produced better outcomes than the approach by the psychiatrist. In addition, I did not really get to discuss things with him. This may have significantly attenuated my worries. After all, he is much more experienced in these issues than I am, and his judgement is certainly superior to mine.

References

Gaynes, B. N., West, S. L., Ford, C. A., Frame, P., Klein, J., Lohr, K. N., and Force, U. P. S. T. (2004). Screening for suicide risk in adults: a summary of the evidence for the US. preventive services task force. *Ann Intern Med*, 140(10):822–835.

Goldsmith, S. K., Pellmar, T. C., Kleinman, A. M., and Bunney, W. E., editors (2003). *Reducing suicide: a national imperative.* Institute of Medicine of the National Academies, The National Academies Press, Washington DC.

Mann, J. J., Apter, A., Bertolote, J., Beautrais, A., Currier, D., Haas, A., Hegerl, U., Lonnqvist, J., Malone, K., Marusic, A., Mehlum, L., Patton, G., Phillips, M., Rutz, W., Rihmer, Z., Schmidtke, A., Shaffer, D., Silverman, M., Takahashi, Y., Varnik, A., Wasserman, D., Yip, P., and Hendin, H. (2005). Suicide prevention strategies: a systematic review. *JAMA*, 294(16):2064–2074.

Oquendo, M. A., Currier, D., and Mann, J. J. (2006). Prospective studies of suicidal behavior in major depressive and bipolar disorders: what is the evidence for predictive risk factors? *Acta Psychiatr Scand*, 114(3):151–158.

COMMENTS ON REFLECTION

This is a good reflective piece that makes enjoyable reading. The author has tried to place himself in the mindset of the patient; he has thought in some detail about how he would feel if he were the patient, what he would have done had he been the psychiatrist and his views about the consultation. He reflects as he narrates and there is a good deal of reflection throughout.

The author has written mainly in the first person, which is a good approach in a reflective piece. The author has also signalled insight into his own inexperience and the general limitations of a psychiatric assessment for patients who have attempted suicide, and shows a mature understanding of medical treatment outcomes in this condition. He expresses his self-doubts courageously and sensibly. The author succeeded in leaving the reader curious and interested in the outcome for this patient; this of course is not a criticism but applause for a good reflective piece.

He mentions his disappointment with the unsatisfactory way the psychiatrist answered his bleep, interrupting the consultation. Instead of criticising here he should apply his obvious insight and ability to reflect-on-action to explore why this might have happened, why the consultant was not at his best and how the consultant may also feel some dissatisfaction.

The piece is a little overlong and the third paragraph and associated references are completely out of place in a reflective piece. While I am sure the author is simply trying to put the situation in context, it is neither core to the description nor evidence of reflection and could be omitted.

COMMENTS ON ENGLISH

What was done well

➤ This essay seems well planned and structured. The student begins with an overview of the situation and the patient, proceeds to detail the situation, explains aspects of suicide and then continues to narrate while reflecting. Whilst the final paragraph seems slightly less focused and a bit "wordy", the student has obviously spent time considering the shape of his essay and thought process, which makes for an enjoyable and engaging reading experience. If you are unsure as to how to plan and structure your account, refer to Figure 2.1.

What could have been done better

➤ A few key words are misspelled, which detracts from the quality of the essay. Errors include "nterest" instead of interest, "nteresting" instead of interesting and "attemped" instead of attempted. Whilst these mistakes seem minor, they can be incredibly irritating to read as they indicate carelessness. If English is not your first language ensure you have a good English dictionary available to you (most online dictionaries are usually reliable) to ensure that your spelling does not let you down. Once you are happy with your draft it is always worth asking a peer who does speak English as a first language to proofread your work for you; at this stage it is a shame to fall victim to poor spelling.

➤ This essay features some "non-sentences". A sentence is a group of words that stand thematically and grammatically independent: every sentence you write must make sense on its own. A straightforward way of checking that your sentence is actually a sentence is by ensuring it includes a verb. The following example includes a "non-sentence" that should actually be incorporated into one of the sentences surrounding it as a subclause. In this situation, colons become particularly useful because words following a colon do not have to make sense independently.

Original student version

I was struck very powerfully by a number of things. First, the situation. I wondered how I would react to it.

Amended version

I was very impressed by a number of things: firstly the situation. I wondered how I would react to it.

Mrs. C sat propped up in her bed on the respiratory ward. A dapper 72 year-old, bent and laid waste by her COPD, her eyes still smiled a greeting at us from behind her oxygen mask; first, on the morning ward round, and later, when she kindly agreed to let me clerk her.

It was clear that Mrs. C was no passive player and that she rather sought to stay in charge of her life and her health. She knew all her medications' names and doses, as she had meticulously self-administered them for years, and she questioned the doctors closely about their treatment plans for her. Three weeks into her hospital stay, she was perfectly groomed, and dressed in her own spotless pyjamas. This attitude was part of the reason that she had managed to cope so well with a succession of medical problems, including a mastectomy for a breast cancer, a thyroidectomy, Parkinson's, and her COPD. The other side to this attitude was that she tended to worry about her health; at the time that I saw her, she was quite anxious, though she tried to hide it.

That evening, I had just started to examine Mrs. C's chest, when her visitor noticed a hospital dispenser with 2 tablets, left on her bedside table. Her visitor first pointed this out to me; she asked me what the tablets were, why they were left on the table, and whether Mrs. C was supposed to have taken them and why no-one had made sure she did so. I replied that I did not know and that we had best check with the nurse. The visitor then showed Mrs. C the tablets; Mrs. C became very upset.

She identified the tablets as her Parkinson's medication; she should have taken them three hours earlier. She said that for fifteen years, she had taken her medication like clockwork, only to come into hospital and be forced to rely entirely on other people who, it seemed, were much more blasé. She became more and more distressed, and said that she would be checking out of the hospital, she'd had enough. She appealed to me, saying "You can see my point, can't you? I'm right, aren't I?"

To which I replied, "Yes, you're right".

I made that reply for several reasons. I had been shocked at finding tablets simply left out like that, as I had thought administering nurses had to watch patients take their medications. More than that, though, I was immersed in Mrs. C's distress. Her health was at stake, and after years of careful effort she had been stripped of control, only for those now in control to fail her through what seemed like sheer carelessness. Faced with Mrs. C's frustration, and her increasingly laboured breathing, I would have agreed with anything she said, because I was desperate to soothe her, and to avoid increasing her agitation by any attempt at an objective response.

Mrs. C's visitor called the nurse in to find out what had happened. Both sides seemed to view me as an adjudicator, each arguing their case to me despite my repeated clarifications that I was just a student and therefore knew the least of anyone in that cubicle. They eventually sorted it through; the nurse apologised and brought fresh tablets. Mrs. C assured the nurse that she didn't blame her per se. However, Mrs. C was still quite wound up and upset by the experience, so much so that she asked me to defer the clerking to the next day.

I left thoroughly disgruntled with myself. I had been aiming to soothe and comfort Mrs. C, to be nice to her in the hope of making her feel better. On the positive side, I think I did establish some rapport with her, and I got her to laugh a bit after the incident. However, on the negative side, I was completely biased in the patient's favour because she was so upset. My objectivity drowned in a flood of compassion, leaving me with no professionalism whatsoever.

I maligned a colleague; as someone affiliated with the hospital and therefore considered by patients to be knowledgeable, I agreed with the patient's criticism of the nurse's conduct before hearing what the nurse had to say.

My overriding motivation was to soothe Mrs. C in any way possible, and to try to cheer her up. I forgot about emotional detachment, professionalism, and keeping my distance. The desire to be a 'nice person', to be almost a friend to the patient, largely overrode my other considerations. Which, I have since come to realise, is profoundly stupid. Patients don't come to hospital just to find people who will be nice to them. They have family and friends for that. Patients don't come to doctors to be mollycoddled. They come because they want to be cured. While in hospital they trust their doctors and nurses precisely because of the rationality, objectivity, detachment and professionalism that are the tenets of the health profession. Patients are ill, scared, and vulnerable; it's almost guaranteed that they will be emotional, and that is exactly why their doctors must never be anything other than level-headed.

This experience made me realise that my attitude to patients is incorrect. As a doctor, my duty to my patients would not consist of attempting to befriend them, as their equal. Rather, my duty will be to place my knowledge and my dispassionate, unemotional critical faculty at their service, in their time of need. That is what I now bear in mind every time I approach a patient; and I hope that this change in my perspective will help me to behave professionally the next time a similar situation arises.

COMMENTS ON REFLECTION

This is good reflection engagingly written. It deals with the rather subtle subject of patient advocacy and doctor–patient relationships.

The reader is brought into the consultation in the first sentence and the description of the patient, her pyjamas and the tablets bring the bedside scenario vividly to life. The author pauses for reflection at each stage, showing thoughtfulness and maturity. The moment when the author answers the patient feels almost like a pause. She has left the reply bald, with no immediate justification for the response, and has created a cliffhanger, where she and the reader know instantly that she thinks she is wrong.

The key thing is that the author reflects on her behaviour, which may or may not have been professional or partisan. Her intuition was correct and she articulates her feelings very well. The author is self-critical in her reflection-on-action, concluding that her "attitude to patients is incorrect", and she shows some rebound emotions about acting more dispassionately and neutrally next time. Remember, though, that doctors are allowed to be emotional. Indeed, cold doctors come across to patients and colleagues as callous, uncaring, robotic and, almost worst of all, disinterested. It is also usually good practice to be "pro-patient" rather than "pro-colleague". The author seems to be the sort of doctor most patients would want if they were ill. Although it could be argued that the student is being overly self-critical, the experience and reflection appear to have made a significant impact on her professional development and she has reflected this in her writing.

COMMENTS ON ENGLISH

What was done well

➤ This essay is written in an interesting and lively way. We all have different voices and we all sound different on paper. Whilst you can admire another person's way of writing, it is almost impossible to adopt their style; developing and maintaining your own personal way of writing is important, particularly in a personal piece of writing such as a reflective essay. You craft your own style through sentence length and vocabulary choices. This student opens her essay with interesting words and phrases such as "propped up", "dapper" and "her eyes still smiled a greeting at us".

➤ This essay is well paragraphed and seems to have been planned carefully as both the situation and the reflection are clearly described and explained. Planning your essay before writing is crucial. If you are unsure as to how to order events or thoughts refer to the flow chart diagram in Chapter 2.

What could have been done better

➤ Although this essay is generally well punctuated, the student is slightly too liberal with her use of commas. Commas should be used to indicate where your reader should pause, to separate one-word items in a list or instead of brackets. Whilst you do not want your sentences to cause your readers a shortage of breath, it is important that you use commas prudently. This student often uses commas unnecessarily and the following examples would benefit from the commas being removed entirely:

Example 1

She knew all her medications' names and doses, as she had meticulously self-administered them for years, and she questioned the doctors closely about their treatment plans for her.

Example 2

Three weeks into her hospital stay, she was perfectly groomed, and dressed in her own spotless pyjamas.

Example 3

My overriding motivation was to soothe Mrs. C in any way possible, and to try to cheer her up.

When considering what to reflect upon for this essay it was clear in my mind which situation has had the greatest impact on me and which has stuck most clearly in my mind and as such was the obvious choice to focus upon. During the first few days of our clinical career myself and the rest of my firm were generally just trying to avoid getting in the way and attempting to settle in as quickly as possible without drawing too much attention to ourselves. It was in this early period, whilst I was still feeling very vulnerable and overwhelmed, that we embarked upon our first ever ward round as part of a firm, in this case as members of the care of the older person firm with Dr. XX. The first few patients went without much ado and as a student I was beginning to settle into the format of the ward round and my expected role. It was at this point that we arrived at the bed of an elderly lady. The patient looked uncomfortable lying on her side and was clinging onto her bedside when we approached and Dr. XX attempted to role her onto her back at which point the patient yelped in pain and started whimpering out for help. The obvious pain she was in was a new site for me and immediately shocked me and I was overwhelmed with a desire to help in some way but of course there was little I could do that was not already being done. As the consultation continued it transpired the patient had very bad infected sores on her ankles which were the source of much of her pain. As Dr. XX continued to sooth the patient and reassure her they would do everything they could to ease the pain the patient closed her eyes and stopped breathing. Dr. XX stopped before looking at us and saying the patient had died. In that moment my emotions were indescribable as a mixture of sadness, shock and pure fear overwhelmed me. After a few moments of silence, during which I felt completely chocked and almost unable to breath, the patient took a deep breath in and then continued to breathe as if nothing has occurred. Obviously shocked by the few seconds that had passed we all stood silent before Dr. XX again reassured the patient that relief from the pain would come before moving out of the cubicle and in our overwhelmed state we followed. Dr. XX then quickly gathered a nurse to contact the daughter who had gone to the cafeteria before addressing the team of doctors to ensure that more morphine was administered. Dr. XX then returned to the patient who was more awake and aware again and assured her that her daughter would be present soon. As we walked away from the patient Dr. XX had been clearly moved and I did see her momentarily wiping away a tear from her eye, a small motion that again pushed my heart into my mouth. The daughter was quickly back on the ward, and after briefly talking to her, Dr. XX left the mother and daughter in peace before resuming the ward round as business-like as before.

For the remainder of the ward round, and in fact the day, I could not remove the huge well of emotions that I was feeling yet could not decipher. Unlike anything I'd felt before I was simply overwhelmed. The obvious pain the patient was in when we first arrived was clear and truly upsetting, seeing another human being in agony begging for help is a horrible thing to deal with. Similarly facing death on a daily basis is a terrible weight to bear. However when actually considering it the sight of a patient in agony and the haunting shadow of death faced day-in-day-out is the reason we become doctors; to help others, to relieve the pain, to fight death and when that is not possible give people the opportunity to say goodbye to their loved ones. Also on that day I realised that it was not only I that had been affected but also the fact Dr. XX wiped away a tear showed me that no matter how long you practice medicine, and no matter how many times a patient is in pain or faces death it is only natural that as a fellow human being you are affected.

COMMENTS ON REFLECTION

This reflective essay describes the clinical scenario well and shows good empathy and high-quality reflection. This is achieved by the style of writing and the use of "I". The subtle and quite powerful description of the consultant's tear and her inter-actions with the family are good and show a significant degree of close observation of what was happening.

The author does not attempt to tell the reader what he would do when witnessing his next death but perhaps his final sentence says it all.

For the purposes of publication we have removed the name of the doctor concerned. The names of patients and colleagues should not be included in reflective pieces without written permission and their inclusion is unnecessary. Comments can be interpreted as defamatory or pejorative even if that is not the author's intention. We have explained our approach of anonymising the submitted essays in our Preface. Although this piece is highly complimentary of a powerful role model, the author is unlikely to have gained the consultant's permission to write about her in such detail.

COMMENTS ON ENGLISH
What was done well
➤ There is some very ambitious vocabulary here that is used, usually accurately and effectively, to convey emotion or circumstance. The key to navigating the fine line between ambitious vocabulary and unnecessary, flowery language is to keep sentences tightly structured and just peppered, not littered, with exciting words and phrases: "It was in this early period, whilst I was still feeling very vulnerable and overwhelmed, that we embarked upon our first ever ward round as part of a firm, in this case as members of the care of the older person firm with Dr. XX." This extract uses a few interesting words such as "vulnerable", "overwhelmed" and "embarked" to extend the meaning of a well-structured sentence.

What could have been done better
➤ The quality of the English is thoroughly let down by poor paragraphing and spelling. These grammatical errors are more than mere glitches; they are major pitfalls that actually frustrate the meaning and clarity of the writing. Paragraph breaks could be inserted to separate the introductory lines that focus the reflection and set it in time: first seeing the patient; the patient's pain; walking away from the patient; and then another paragraph for reflecting. Separating each episode into a paragraph focuses writing and gives it a sense of movement and development.
➤ This essay is a classic example of how erroneous a computer spellcheck can be. Spellcheck is mechanical and cannot interpret meaning or purpose. It did not

detect "role" for "roll", "soothe", "choked" or "shocked" for "chocked". Sloppy spelling errors are easy for a tutor to spot and show unsatisfactory proofreading and lack of attention to detail, which are major defects in a doctor. Having written your essay, don't let yourself down by ignoring its presentation to your reader who will be judging you and your approach to your course. A good way of eliminating these errors from your work is to ask a friend to read your work over. Often a different set of eyes can spot errors that you have missed.

Since starting clinical medicine in September of this year I have been faced with many situations that caused me to reflect upon what it means to be a doctor and how best to treat and respect patients. Circumstances arise almost every day where a decision could have been made differently, a patient could have been treated more fairly or a particular doctor has stuck in my mind for being impressive in his or her treatment of patients.

I was on a haematology ward round with a consultant a registrar and two SHOs. I had noticed at other times when being on this particular ward that one of the patients liked to come out of his side room and wander around the ward, I had also been told that he may be confused and could act unpredictably or inappropriately. In a discussion with an SHO earlier on in the week she told me that over the weekend shift he had got particularly agitated and at one point had to be physically restrained. During the ward round I had noticed him, as usual, wandering around. As we were in the corridor discussing one of the patients we were interrupted by some of the nurses shouts and a commotion coming from round the corner. We then saw the patient in question come round the corner grabbing hold of the security guard and hitting him repeatedly. This obviously shocked me and I turned to the other doctors for some indication of how to react. It seemed at this point that no-one was really sure what to do, the patient was very aggressively hitting and kicking the security guard and pushed him all the way down the corridor past where we were standing. The guard was trying to stop him and obviously did not want to hurt the patient but was himself bleeding from his nose and obviously injured. At this point one of the SHOs ran off to get help, and the registrar, who knew the patient, attempted to calm him down. Eventually she was able to calm the patient and take him back to his room and the security guard was able to go and get his injuries checked over. Later I was up on the ward again checking a patients notes, the ward was full of security and doctors discussing how to manage the patient and one of the nurses came over to talk to me. "You were there when it happened weren't you? Still want to be a doctor?" he joked. He then told me that the doctors were planning to sedate the patient to be able to give him treatment as he was potentially a danger to himself and others. "I told them they should do this days ago" he said "the patient has been like this for a while".

This incident really affected me not just because it was shocking and I felt scared for myself and the other people involved, but because it also made me think about how difficult it is to manage a patient like this, whilst still treating him with respect and dignity. It made me think about the balance between doing the best for the patient and making sure the staff and people around him are safe. Immediately as the incident happened I felt for both the patient and obviously the security guard, but for myself I almost felt redundant, helpless. I didn't know what I should do and to this day don't really know what would have been the right actions to take, so I just stood there and watched it happen. Maybe I could have done more, but what exactly I don't know. I certainly was not the right person to get involved to try to stop the fight and I did not know the patient well enough to try and calm him down.

After the event my thoughts really turned to the patient. From talking to the doctors I understand that he was not an aggressive man before and must be really quite ill to have got into the state he is in. He had multiple medical problems and is on a lot of medication. It is very sad for him that the only option left is to sedate him, and I wonder whether there is really nothing else that can be done for him. I guess in the end the safety of not just everyone around him but the patient himself is the most important thing, and that if sedating him is the only way to give him the treatment that will make him well again, then it is in his best interest for the doctors to do this.

There was one thing that particularly impressed me during this incident and that is the actions of the registrar. She acted calmly and always with the best interests of the patient in mind. She managed to almost single-handedly calm the patient down without having to use any physical restraint and with seemingly no worry for her own safety. I think that if a situation similar to this should arise in the future I will think of the actions of this doctor and try to act the same myself.

On reflection of the event I think that that probably taking no action may have been the best action to take. I was not experience or trained enough to be able to deal with the situation and getting myself involved may have done more harm then good. I think though that I could have acted quicker in going to get help and in supporting the other doctors that were there, and I would aim to do this in the future.

COMMENTS ON REFLECTION

This essay contains some rather superficial, instantaneous shock reflection rather than a comprehensive analysis of this rather frightening experience. The author appears to be mainly concerned with defending her inactivity rather than exploring in more detail how she felt, what it meant to her, the medical aspects of the case and whether she could and should have played a more active role from which she would probably have learned much more. Passive observation in medicine at the undergraduate stage is normal but not always necessary and certainly not enough to gain valuable experience. It is disappointing that we are not told why the patient was violent and what the underlying diagnosis was. One hopes the author discussed the medical aspects of the case with the medical team to find out why the patient was violent because clinical management is directed at the cause, although protecting the patient and the clinical staff is the first priority. A more rounded reflection might also include more than emotions and the author could have included a reflection on the medical aspects of this case.

The author did not tell the reader how she felt when the nurse asked her if she still wanted to be a doctor. This would have been an excellent issue to reflect upon. Also how did she feel about the nurse's view that this episode could have been prevented if the patient had been sedated earlier?

The author concluded that she was correct in not getting involved because she would not have known what to do, but is this correct? Doctors at all stages of their careers will face unfamiliar and unsettling experiences that they have to manage without formal training or previous clinical exposure. Initiative, common sense and the ability to think through, act and respond to clinical situations is a fundamentally important attribute of doctors. Patients have high and often unrealistic expectations of doctors. Standing back and observing a violent patient and the actions of others is easier than helping the patient and other staff cope with the problem. There was no reason why the author could not have offered to help the staff and get involved. It might have been a much more educational experience for her.

The author's conclusion that her inaction was the best course of action is not persuasive and she appears to have reached this conclusion after the efficient intervention by the registrar. This suggests that there was no major organic problem with the patient who may have been frightened or antagonised by the security guard. She does not discuss what she could and would have done had she been alone with the patient, although she reflected that she would have tried to act like the registrar; this is not always possible. If, in future, she is confronted with a similar situation with an uncooperative patient, what did she learn from this experience that would help her? What medical aspects of the violent or confused patient did she learn?

COMMENTS ON ENGLISH

What was done well

➤ This essay begins with a very good introduction that concisely reflects upon the student's medical experiences in general and then leads on seamlessly to the specific incident upon which they are reflecting. Whilst introductions are not totally necessary in a piece of reflective writing, a series of succinct sentences that introduce and justify your topic can be an effective starting point.
➤ The sentences in this essay are mostly well constructed and appear to be simply phrased, making the work very easy to read; this is a sign of good written English.

What could have been done better

➤ It is clear that this student is not aware of how to use apostrophes correctly and a few possessive apostrophes have been omitted from this piece of work. Possessive apostrophes must be inserted where appropriate as without them meaning can be changed or even lost. (*See* punctuation section in Chapter 2 for details on appropriate use of apostrophes.) The first example requires a possessive apostrophe, although, arguably, one can understand the sentence without it as the patient is referred to as "a patient" (that is, one patient). The second example from this essay also requires a possessive apostrophe; however, unlike the first example it is very difficult, if not impossible, to make sense of, as the reader is unsure whether the sentence refers to a single nurse or a group of nurses.

Original student version

Later I was up on the ward again checking a patients notes, the ward was full of security and doctors discussing how to manage the patient and one of the nurses came over to talk to me.

Amended version

Later I was up on the ward again checking a patient's notes. The ward was full of security and doctors discussing how to manage the patient and one of the nurses came over to talk to me.

Original student version

As we were in the corridor discussing one of the patients we were interrupted by some of the nurses shouts and a commotion coming from round the corner.

Amended version

As we were in the corridor discussing one of the patients we were interrupted by some of the nurse's shouts and a commotion coming from round the corner.

I walk tentatively into cubicle 5, Accident and Emergency, on the second day of my critical care placement. Shes young, probably only a few years older than me. She looks exhausted and pain is etched across her face. As I prepare the equipment for cannulation, that familiar feeling of dread creeps over me. This isn't going to work. I'm not going to hit the vein. I'm going to hurt her...and I still won't get that plastic tube inside her. Deep breaths, look confident, smile re-assuringly. "Hi, my name is X, I'm a third year medical student...". She looks a little unconviced, but my supervisor provides some comforting words and she agrees. She tells me shes scared of needles. Oh god. I take her arm, fumble at the tourniquet, and search for that perfect juicy vein. After a quick swab, I warn her of a "sharp scratch". I look up once before I push it in and give her a smile – I'm trying to re-assure her, make her feel comfortable. I wonder though, am I just trying to re-assure myself? Hoping to see her smiling back at me, completely at ease. No luck – she looks terrified. In goes the needle. Flashback? No. My heart sinks. After three years of pre-clinical lectures, tutorials and examinations – this feeling of repeated failiure is alien to me. My supervisor kneels down next to me and attempts to assist, to replace the cannula, but without success. I can't quite turn his suggestions into any form of useful action. I become very aware of the writhing patient beside me and let go of the needle so that he can put her out of her misery. I step back as he applies pressure to the site, and prepares for a second attempt.

I've been here before. Feeling useless, guilty and annoyed at the side. Its a horrible feeling, I may not have put her life in danger, but I hate feeling that I've put her through uneccessary pain. Medicine often inflicts pain, but when a doctor or nurse does it, it is fruitful. I know that one day that will be me, that it will suddenly all fall into place, that even if I'm not successful the first time round, I'll understand why and will have the confidence and skill to quickly and calmly rectify the problem. Until then however, I'm left feeling utterly disheartened.

I've had this conversation with myself before, and its at this point I realise that its a pointless one. I will remember these failed attempts for many weeks, but for this young woman in front of me, in a few days time, these first hours in hospital will probably be nothing but a blur of uncertainty, anxiety and fear. As my supervisor re-gathers the equipment I edge closer to the bed and reach out to hold the gauze over her arm where my needle had been. I catch her eye and try to convey, somehow, that I'm sorry. I want to make it okay. I know you're scared. I rub her arm and give it a squeeze. She looks up and smiles. I think shes grateful. Within a few seconds the cannula is in, the dressing is on, and we are clearing our things.

On reflection, it made me acknowlege how powerful the gesture of holding a patients hand, of rubbing their arm, of looking them in the eye, can be. We spend days on the ward examining patients and hours in surgery elbow deep in their bowels and though this contact is healing, it is ultimately clinical, and will be felt as such by the patient. I remember my grandmothers recent stay in hospital – the nurses who didn't care, the doctors who never addressed her. This was her story, and its one that I've heard time and time again in newspapers and round the dinner table. It saddens me that she felt this way, because my experience of clinical medicine has been, on the whole, a positive one. The vast majority of staff care deeply about their patients, although they often seem worn down by the system within which they work. My grandmothers experience, and mine that day as I tried to cannulate the young woman, illustrates to me how *feeling* alone is not enough, how instead, we must actively communicate these inner thoughts to the patient.

I once read that "people will forget what you said, people will forget what you did, but people will never forget how you made them feel". Nowhere is this more evident than in medicine. My 90 year old grandmother left hospital within a week; tired, bruised, but essentially "cured" despite being very ill at one point; clearly, the doctors and nurses did their job. Surprisingly though, my grandmother felt little gratitude towards them. The only person she consistently spoke well of was an FY1 who she recalled by name. He came to see her every day, to ask how she was doing, have a little chat. He was the same FY1 who was responsible for the bruises exending almost from shoulder to wrist due to repeated botched blood tests and cannulation attempts on her frail arm.

Its then that you realise that no matter how successful (or unsuccessful) you may be in addressing the patients medical needs, a small gesture of humanity is what the patient needs to feel that you care. To know that you care. I truly hope that the woman I tried, and failed to cannulate, remembers me not as the medical student who gave her that massive bruise on her hand, but as the person who gave her a smile, who tried to understand, as much as I could, how frightened she must have been feeling, and wanted to make it better.

COMMENTS ON REFLECTION

This is good reflection. A very personal, empathic, mature and sensitive account of cannulation. The author has captured the fear and lack of confidence felt by novices and also some senior doctors when doing practical procedures.

The reflection shows both reflection-in-action and reflection-on-action and an ability to mesh the thoughts and feelings that were aroused with what the author already knew to be true but which has now been reinforced by the encounter.

Cannulation and phlebotomy are very popular choices for reflective writing for students new to workplace-based learning. Although they are good choices your reader has read very similar pieces many times before. You might try to think of another powerful event if you want your reflection to catch the eye of the reader.

COMMENTS ON ENGLISH

What was done well

➤ The style of this essay is interesting and engaging. A lot of this essay is written in the present tense, which is unusual but effective in this case as it creates a sense of intimacy and urgency; it allows the reader to empathise with the writer as the distance between situation, writer and reader is bridged. However, it is key that you write in a style that most suits you. It is very obvious when someone tries to write in a style they have seen somewhere else but are not totally comfortable with themselves. When they do, this may result in errors. You should try and write in a style that comes naturally to you. This will usually allow you to produce the most persuasive and readable English which should sound sensible and convincing.

What could have been done better

➤ This essay is full of careless spelling and grammatical mistakes. Whilst the errors are relatively minor, their frequency detracts from the overall quality of the work. Whilst no one will shoot you down for forgetting one apostrophe or comma, repeatedly making the same mistakes throughout an extended piece of work could thoroughly test the nerves and patience of your reader. Careful proofreading, reading the essay aloud with a friend or into a Dictaphone or even using the spellcheck on your computer in a sensible, objective way can easily reduce the level of such mistakes in your work.

➤ The student repeatedly writes "shes" which is not a word at all and is actually an abbreviation of "she is". The correct version is "she's". The apostrophe replaces the missing "i". The word "its" is also repeatedly used incorrectly to the same effect. The student writes "Its a horrible feeling" when they should have written "It is a horrible feeling". Whilst it is preferable to avoid abbreviations in formal academic work, you will not get heavily penalised for using them as long as you use them properly.

➤ The student has also misspelled key words such as "exending" instead of "extending" and "acknowlege" instead of "acknowledge". If in doubt, you should always check important spellings with a dictionary. These look like careless attempts at writing and laziness in not reading through and checking spelling, for which there is no excuse!

Choosing the topic for this reflective piece proved very difficult. Thorough the four- plus months we have spent learning in hospital I have seen and done many things which I am sure will stick with me through my life, though I will almost certainly experience them many times over. The nature of 3rd year medicine- the uncertainty of what we are doing, the lack of practice, the worry that we will cause irreversible harm through our own incompetence is what I believe to both drives and terrify most students. For myself, one event clearly sticks out in my mind where the sum of all those fears was realised; assisting in a cardiac arrest on A&E.

Two weeks before I was to end Gen Med myself and another student from my firm had gone down to A&E in the middle of the day, with the idea of practising cannulation. We walked into a fairly empty resus room, at which time the call went out announcing a patient in cardiac arrest was minutes away. I remember looking at the team which had gathered to attempt to save the patients life. It looked too small compared to those I had seen during night shifts on A&E. One of the doctors saw me and asked me to do chest compressions on the patient when he came in. This was probably one of the most terrifying moments in my life.

While jogging over to the resus bay, attempting to pull my gloves on my mind was a incoherent mess. I blanked completely on the teaching we have on the introductory course in medicine regarding BLS. How many compressions a minute am I meant to do? How deep? Oddly I did recall the notions I had head about how chest compressions break ribs. Probably unhelpful at that point. I vividly recall one of the nurses handing me a pair of gloves, telling me that I had to wear them. I was startled out of my stupor and began pulling on the gloves. Adrenaline pumping and sweating, my hand tore straight through the first one before I managed to get a hand into the other glove. Then the paramedics wheeled the patient in.

I remember looking at the patient, a man I thought could be no older than 60, with endotracheal tube already in place and chest compressions being done by one of the paramedics. They wheeled the patient next to the bed where we were all standing, myself still with only one glove on. We lifted the patient to the bed and I immediately began chest compressions. I remember getting complete tunnel vision at this point. All I recall the small square of the patient's chest I was pounding on, keeping count to the song "staying alive" as taught during the introductory course. The feel of the chest under my hands was so strange. It just felt wrong to be pushing so hard on an actual person compared to the models we were so briefly taught on.

After two minutes of chest compressions had passed I was instructed to stop, so peripheral pulses could be checked. It was at this point the nurse told me to put on another glove. I was aghast. 'Does that really matter right now?' It seemed so inappropriate to me to think about infection control and good practise to what was my mind having the patient's life in my hands. The rest of the team did not see it from my point of view, so while one of the paramedics took over while I put a glove on the remaining hand. I think it was at this moment that I stopped and began to think about what was happening more clearly. The team I was with had probably done dozens of these and would stop me if I was doing anything wrong. They also knew what was needed to be done to try and save the patient. I was now working as a member of that team. I realised that the patient's life was not really in my hands. The team was working against the odds to try to save the patient. I had my role to play as a member of that team and so had to focus on that role and push away all the emotions. Strangely, that realisation seemed to quell the panic I felt. For the next

8 minutes we preformed the ALS algorithm, but unfortunately we could not resuscitate the patient.

After we stopped, I remember looking at the colleague we came in with and recognising the same panic I had and still felt. One of the doctors came up to me afterwards and asked 'first time?', while nodding sympathetically. I remember asking him if there was anything that we could have done. In actuality, I wanted to know that I had not made a mistake. He told me how the patient had come in without any heart beat and he had never seen someone recover from that. He told me that what I had done was correct and thanked me. While very much shocked at what I had experienced I also felt grateful for those few words which got rid of that ill- directed worry that I had somehow been at fault.

Astonishingly 3 weeks later I was again asked to perform chest compressions on a patient on A&E, although there were many more people around this time. I was shocked at the difference the first experience had in me. Having dwelt on the first occasion and learnt from it. I felt calm and focussed compared to the sheer panic and anxiety I experienced first time. I do not believe I will ever be able to readily accept deaths in these circumstances, but I know now that to blame oneself unnecessarily is a fatal misconception for a medical student.

COMMENTS ON REFLECTION

There is reflection in this piece but not much. The vast majority is reflection-in-action and while some of it is good quality the author could have done more. For example, he tells us "This was probably one of the most terrifying moments in my life" but does not tell us why. He did not reflect on the value or ethics of resuscitating a patient who had "come in without any heart beat". Did the author understand this and what he was trying to do? What did he learn about resuscitation, the role of students and other staff in resuscitation?

The author seems to have learned that many clinical procedures and events are difficult on the first occasion but become less intimidating and difficult on subsequent occasions. However, when describing his second attempt he simply says, "Having dwelt on the first occasion and learnt from it" but gives the reader no indication of what he learned and why.

It is extremely important to get the words "practise" the verb, and "practice" the noun, right *all* the time.

COMMENTS ON ENGLISH
What was done well

➤ This essay is well paragraphed. Each paragraph marks a development in the story or a shift in perspective and the work is therefore easy for a reader to digest.
➤ The student has varied sentence length for effect; important revelations are articulated in short, sharp sentences to create a powerful effect: "This was probably one of the most terrifying moments in my life."

What could have been done better

➤ There are a few different types of grammatical errors in this piece of work and these could have been remedied with careful proofreading. It is extremely obvious when work has not been carefully proofread as mistakes, such as using the wrong punctuation mark, inconsistent verb and noun agreements, and unnecessary words let down an otherwise clear essay. The following sentence exemplifies most of these issues:

Original student version

The nature of 3rd year medicine- the uncertainty of what we are doing, the lack of practice, the worry that we will cause irreversible harm through our own incompetence is what I believe to both drives and terrify most students.

Amended version

There are several challenges facing third-year students; our uncertainty of what we are doing, our lack of practice, experience and knowledge, and our anxieties that we will cause irreversible harm through our incompetence both drive and terrify most of us.

A number of changes have been made in the improved version and they appear in detail below:

1 Writing numbers as letters: in academic essays it is always preferable to write "third year" as opposed to "3rd year".
2 The use of a colon: the dash has been replaced with a colon. Dashes are slightly too informal for academic work and in this case a colon is more appropriate as they are used to introduce a list of items.
3 The use of semicolons: semicolons have replaced commas; they herald a longer pause than commas and are more appropriate for separating longer items on a list.
4 Practise and practice: the former is a verb, the latter a noun. The verb, practise, should be used in this instance as the student is referring to the action of practising, rather than the absence or lack of patients in his personal practice. For example, a doctor may have a busy practice that keeps him practising long hours.
5 Nouns and verbs agreeing: it is important that nouns and verbs agree. If you write about "a patient" you would write "he feels" but if you were writing about "patients" you would write "they feel". Note how the singular or plural endings of the verb must agree with the plural or singular noun respectively. The improved version therefore reads: "drives and terrifies" instead of "drives and terrify".
6 Unnecessary words: proofreading should always involve some pruning of the word count. Unnecessary words can often bog down the reader by congesting sentences and this clogs the meaning of your essay. The words "is what I believe to" have been removed in the improved version as they are superfluous. A reflective essay is personal; the author is writing about only his beliefs.

For this exercise I have chosen a patient who came in by ambulance on the night I was on take in December 2007. The call that had come out was that a young, possibly Kurdish man had taken a very serious overdose of tricyclic antidepressants and the paramedics had found him unresponsive and fitting. The patient arrived in the resuscitation room and after several cycles of CPR, he died. It was revealed during the resuscitation that the man was only 21 years old and had been brought in after phoning one of the few people he knew in London to inform him he had taken 90 of these tablets which was six times the normal lethal dose.

Reflection
This had been my busiest night on take. It had been a very useful night from a learning perspective and I had also enjoyed the experience. This case though had many different aspects that I needed to reflect upon.

Firstly, although this was not the first patient to have died while I was on the crash team, it was the first time I had witnessed the death of someone younger than me die. I would have expected to have found the situation more harrowing at the time but I think I sufficed myself by honestly knowing that each of the 10 people at the scene had used all their training and expertise to help this boy. The fact was that he had taken 90 of these tablets, he had been suffering from depression for a long time and it was not his first attempt at suicide strongly implied that he wanted to end his life that night.

The most worrying thing was my detachment from the situation. The first time I had seen someone die in the resuscitation room had been quite traumatic and this time, it made me think that I had subconsciously already developed the skill of detachment. While this is an almost inevitable 'skill' for junior doctors acquire, it does make one feel that one had lost a part of that empathetic character many were so proud of at medical school interviews. The fact remained that there was nothing more medically that could have been done and I honestly believed that the boy had wanted to end his life that night. I felt for the helplessness of the boy's situation but also felt pretty helpless as a medic because 10 fully trained personal with all the technology and science available to them, still could not restart the rhythm of those fibrillating ventricles.

This brings me on to my second area of reflection: it was the first time that I had seen someone die from a suicide attempt. The history would imply that the boy really had wanted to end his life that night. I certainly believed that the night he died and immediately had tremendous sympathy for his situation, which must have been so very desperate. The decision to take one's own life however is never one taken lightly and it is such a violent and terminating decision to make that it is one that could be argued, can never be made by anyone unless they are in an irrational state of mind. The argument as to whether someone has the right to commit suicide or not is however separate to the decision about the level of care that should be provided to someone that has made a serious attempt at suicide. It would seem logical that someone who had decided to commit suicide would have also not consented to medical treatment to reverse their decision. This argument does nevertheless rely very heavily on the fact that the patient really did want to end their life and without any documentary, very solid evidence that this was in fact the case, it would be a brave doctor who did not offer assistance in this scenario.

The crash calls are made and the whole team, including the students, goes into a rehearsed mode of advanced life support. There did not seem to be any consideration of the boy's wishes or desires. There was no evidence of his beliefs or requests but it is unlikely he wanted to see out his final night with me clumsily attempting to insert large bore canulas into his forearms and later compressing his chest with all the force I could muster at 2am. It certainly is not a dignified way to leave the World but he may also have appreciated our last final efforts. If saving life is our primary objective, it would appear that our chance would have passed many months before that night is December.

The situation of a 21 year old refugee committing suicide just before Christmas was a very emotional experience especially as my hands were still on him when the decision was made to stop the resuscitation. It may have brought out too many emotions to write about in just one piece but it has certainly highlighted the importance of reflecting upon these situations so that one may better understand the role and limitations of a doctor.

COMMENTS ON REFLECTION

This is a powerful and well-written story but there is actually little personal reflection here. There is a paragraph on the ethics of suicide but the author unfortunately discusses the events as an onlooker rather than telling us how he felt about the patient's presentation, the circumstances and his role in the attempted resuscitation. The essay is mainly a discussion of the ethics and philosophy of suicide. The author explains his "detachment" when witnessing his first suicide, justifying it with his belief that the patient wanted to end his life and that there was nothing he could do, and his belief that the patient would have refused treatment or resuscitation. Is this a loss of empathy or resignation and, if so, is this something that he thinks is a helpful coping mechanism? The author states that "it may have brought out too many emotions to write about" but he did not truly attempt to write about any of them, other than finally stating that it is important to reflect "upon these situations". The author does not let us know how he will feel about the next death he witnesses or the next successful or unsuccessful suicide. What did the author learn, and how did it help his professional development?

COMMENTS ON ENGLISH

What was done well

➤ This essay is written in an interesting and lively way. Whilst the account isn't hugely detailed, it is generally interesting and enjoyable to read. Good extracts include the following sentences that are relatively enjoyable to read:

I felt for the helplessness of the boy's situation but also felt pretty helpless as a medic because 10 fully trained personal with all the technology and science available to them, still could not restart the rhythm of those fibrillating ventricles.

There was no evidence of his beliefs or requests but it is unlikely he wanted to see out his final night with me clumsily attempting to insert large bore canulas into his forearms and later compressing his chest with all the force I could muster at 2am.

What could have been done better

➤ This essay would have benefited from some careful proofreading, by either the student or a peer, as certain words are used erroneously and misspelled (personal rather than personnel). Whilst it is important to be ambitious with your vocabulary, you must ensure that you know the meaning of the words you use and you use the right words in the right places. If you are unsure whether you are using a word correctly, check in a dictionary or thesaurus, or ask someone who knows. If a sentence sounds clumsy or is difficult to understand, it probably is. Read it aloud, cut out unnecessary words, rewrite it until the sentence is clear and simple and something that you would have no difficulty saying to someone.

In the following example, the word "sufficed" has been used erroneously:

Original student version

I would have expected to have found the situation more harrowing at the time but I think I sufficed myself by honestly knowing that each of the 10 people at the scene had used all their training and expertise to help this boy.

Amended version

I would have expected to have found the situation more harrowing at the time but I was comforted knowing that each of the 10 people at the scene had used all their training and expertise to help this boy.

"The dehumanising effect of illness on the patient and the consequent problems of autonomy, consent and best interest"

People do not often attend accident and emergency out of choice, but rather through necessity. Doctors often observe people at their most ill, vulnerable and even inhuman state. By human state, I mean a functioning human state, of action and thought. Particularly challenging is a patient for which such a nadir in functioning is likely to be progressive and non reversible because of a lack of efficacious treatment.

Ms. X an MS sufferer in her thirties. I saw her in the accident and emergency department during an on take. She was acutely unwell; she was not alert and was suspected to be pyrexic and dehydrated because of an infection. The patient, although tacitly responsive to verbal commands did not speak, and appeared ill and restless. I was asked to take blood from this patient for FBC, U&Es, LFTs and blood cultures. The patient wore adult nappies, which were assumed to be a result of her MS. The carer was not present, so ascertaining what level of functioning or understanding the patient had when well was not possible to determine. For informed consent of adult information must be able to be understood, retained and weighed. Non coercion is another requisite as is the ability to communicate one's wishes. The default assumption for an adult is competence, and after questioning it became clear that the patient concerned was not competent to give consent for this particular procedure.

When incompetent patients may have made advanced decisions on health care or given a person lasting power of attorney whilst competent. Both of which have statutory backing as outlined in the Mental Capacity Act 2005.

No such indications were present in this case to direct doctors.

In this situation it was deemed that taking the blood was in the patient's best interest. I explained the procedure as simply as I could and then attempted to take the blood, which was unsuccessful. The patient became unhappy, so a nurse performed the procedure. The nurse was ultimately successful after a few attempts, but it was clear that the patient was distressed during the final attempts. The patient did not understand the reasons behind why we were inflicting momentary pain i.e. the needle to take blood. Despite understanding the reasoning behind carrying on with the investigation, it did not make observing the patient's discomfort particularly easy.

Autonomy seems to be central to all consent. But if the doctors had respected the patient's non verbal communications and ultimately respected the patient's autonomy, the blood would not have been taken and the patient would be at risk of a severe infection. When a patient is not competent it seems autonomy is no longer the central issue rather best interests. What would be best for the patient taking into account all that is known about the patient?

In this case very little was known of the patient's character. I think on reflection that putting increased emphasis on contacting family, friends or the patient's GP before commencement of investigations would have been useful. Although I did not anticipate failing to take blood, in such a potentially difficult case, I could have deferred to somebody more experienced with a higher chance of immediate success to minimise discomfort for the patient.

Aside from my concerns over the patient's ability to give informed consent, the situation highlighted other important aspects of healthcare.

Investigations and treatments are rarely without discomfort or side effect. Although the sharp scratch of a needle during venesection may not be hugely detrimental, the act of inflicting pain is not easy for somebody who wishes to alleviate suffering.

Acting in a person's best interests requires doctors to try and think as the patient concerned. This task had seemed relatively straightforward, but I imagine where the evidence for intervention is less strong, such decisions would be very difficult, even if an accurate and detailed portrait of the patient were available.

The image of a young person unable to speak or move as they wished and incontinent was quite obviously difficult. Standing next to her, unable to know what her usual level of functioning was, my mind naturally performed the different iterations possible. The possibility of her requiring help to eat, bath, leave the house. Although there are of course disease modifying drugs for MS, no cure is available. As a potential health care professional I must face up to the reality that I will not be able to help some people as much as I would like.

COMMENTS ON REFLECTION

This is a very poor piece of reflective writing and it seems to stem from the author's lack of understanding (or perhaps refusal to engage with) the nature and very purpose of reflective writing. The rather grand title, the unsubstantiated statements and overambitious language in the opening paragraph, together with the completely unnecessary information about the Mental Capacity Act, is not a good start for a piece of reflective writing. The unclear description and the total lack of reflection that follows do not improve things. The language and tense used does not help the author; for example: "In this situation it was deemed that taking the blood was in the patient's best interest". Deemed by whom and on what assumptions? The reader is left without any indication of what the author has learned from the situation and how this has helped them in their professional growth.

COMMENTS ON ENGLISH

What was done well

➤ This student has used ambitious vocabulary with varying degrees of accuracy. Some sentences are well constructed and effectively articulated, such as: "Although the sharp scratch of a needle during venesection may not be hugely detrimental, the act of inflicting pain is not easy for somebody who wishes to alleviate suffering". This sentence is worded precisely and easy to follow: there are no unnecessary words here as each word adds meaning.

What could have been done better

➤ Whilst vocabulary is varied and ambitious in places, the student actually often overcomplicates sentences with flowery language, which obscures meaning. Precision and accuracy in writing is key: if you wouldn't say it aloud, you shouldn't write it down.

Original student version

Doctors often observe people at their most ill, vulnerable and even inhuman state. By human state, I mean a functioning human state, of action and thought. Particularly challenging is a patient for which such a nadir in functioning is likely to be progressive and non reversible because of a lack of efficacious treatment.

Amended version
Doctors regularly encounter patients who may have physical and/or mental disabilities and are therefore vulnerable. Treatment of such patients is challenging.

➤ Poor punctuation and grammar affect the quality of this essay. Non-sentences include: "Ms. X an MS sufferer in her thirties." A sentence must have a verb (an action word or "doing word" that may often, but not always, end with the suffix "ing") in order to make sense on its own. Without a verb, a sentence is simply a phrase or a clause. An improved version could read: "Ms. X was an MS sufferer in her thirties." Simply adding the verb "was" enables the phrase to mean something independently and become a sentence.

➤ Some sentences are also poorly punctuated, which hinders meaning; for example: "Autonomy seems to be central to all consent. But if the doctors had respected the patient's non verbal communications and ultimately respected the patient's autonomy, the blood would not have been taken and the patient would be at risk of a severe infection." These two sentences should have been linked: the word "but" is a connective and should never be used to begin a sentence (a similar rule applies to the words "and" and "because"). The student could have linked these two sentences by simply removing the full stop before the word "but".

➤ The essay is also poorly paragraphed. The paragraph breaks appear arbitrary when they should actually mirror changes in time, idea or subject. Whilst paragraphs must be well linked, they must be manipulated carefully to split the essay effectively.

There have been many occasions over the past couple of months when I have reflected on my experiences during the General Medicine rotation, however one particular experience has stood out. Whilst on the Respiratory attachment I attended a ward round which was led by a consultant. The team initially spoke for an hour in a meeting room discussing each patient before the actual ward round began. I listened carefully and tried to remember what condition each patient had, however once the actual ward round began I found myself forgetting the patients' details. Midway through the ward round we went to see an 82-year-old female. She appeared in some distress. The consultant approached the patient, introduced himself and asked how the patient was. The patient kept muttering "Not good, not good" and then punched the consultant in the face. I remember being completely stunned and wasn't sure how the consultant would react. The consultant then said in a calm voice "Please don't do that" and asked again how the patient was. The patient again tried to hit the consultant who this time, expecting the punch, caught the patient's hands. He waited a few moments and whilst holding her arms then asked in a clam voice whether there was anything he could do to help her. The patient replied, "Go away!" The consultant asked a few more times whether there was anything he could do to help, but the patient kept replying "Go away!" Having spent in total 3-4 minutes in the room, we all left. Once I got outside I remembered from the meeting before the ward round that this lady had bipolar disorder and due to her current medical condition, she was unable to take her bipolar disorder medication (thus providing further explanation for the previous event).

Later that day I spent time reflecting on the experience. I was initially stunned, as I had never seen a patient attack a member of the health staff. This experience got me thinking about how I would react to a patient physically attacking me, whether or whether not the patient had a psychotic condition (and therefore not in complete control of their actions). Before this experience I think I would have probably left the room straight away to protect myself from further injury. I would not have raised my voice, however I think I would have probably said in a clam voice that violence is not acceptable, and that if the patient continued I would be unable to help them. I believe that health staff have a right to protect themselves and so leaving, unless there was an emergency, would be a reasonable thing to do. However the consultant did not react like this, and in fact I was extremely impressed by how the consultant handled the situation. The consultant knew the lady had bipolar disorder and may not have been taken her medication, however he was definitely shocked when he was punched. He stayed calm, and rather than leaving straight away, he stayed to see if the patient would calm down and whether he could help in any way. He stayed in the room for 3 minutes after being hit, hoping that he would be able to help. If the patient was sound of mind, and had turned violent because they were angry, I'm not sure how he would have reacted.

The General Medical Council say that the duties of a doctor include making the care of the patient your first concern and that all patients should be treated politely and considerately. The consultant definitely made the care of the patient his first concern, even at risk of physical harm, and was still considerate even after being punched. The question can be asked that is the care of the patient more important than the safety of the health staff?

Although I feel that the consultant handled this particular situation very well, I do feel that each situation has to be assessed individually and the risk of physical harm has to be evaluated appropriately. I do not feel that a doctor has to put himself in significant harm. The patient in question was an elderly woman in a bed who couldn't really cause much physical harm. The consultant quickly evaluated whether he had significant risk of physical harm and decided that the risk was very low. Additionally I feel that in this situation, the patient was not in complete control of her actions, and did not have proper intent to cause damage, it was more of a 'leave me alone' punch. If however the patient had been able to cause more harm (perhaps by being very physically strong or in possession of an object, which could have been used as a weapon) or had real intent to cause damage, then perhaps leaving the room sooner would have been advised, and maybe even having the patient restrained would have been necessary.

If in the future I am physically harmed, I hope that after this experience I would quickly assess the situation, evaluating the danger to the patient, myself, other patients and other health staff, and take appropriate action, whether that's staying with the patient - hoping they will calm down, leaving the room right away, or even having the patient restrained.

COMMENTS ON REFLECTION

The author describes the clinical scene vividly and clearly, and we are made to feel shocked and scared by the patient. Assaults against health workers are a problem and not at all easy to deal with. When assaulted, most students, doctors and nurses would feel fear and anger in the same way as if they had been assaulted outside the hospital. Things are slightly different, however, if the assailant is a psychotic patient in hospital. Being assaulted by someone who needs help is one of the biggest challenges in doctor–patient interactions, and requires skill and experience.

It is good that this episode has encouraged the author to think about what it would be like for her if she were to be assaulted. The author is obviously impressed by the ability of the consultant to deal with the event and tries to unpick how she was able to respond in this way. There is, however, not a very deep level of personal reflection anywhere in the account. We are told what she thinks she would do if a similar event happened to her, but this is not explored further.

COMMENTS ON ENGLISH
What was done well
➤ This piece of writing is of an acceptable quality. It is well structured and although the last paragraph is only one sentence long, the other paragraph breaks are well measured and purposeful, which indicates good planning.

What could have been done better
➤ This essay includes some unnecessary brackets. Whilst brackets are perfectly useable punctuation marks, they are often inappropriate in formal academic essays as they break sentences up and distract the reader. Bracketing commas

are preferable to brackets in such pieces of work; they function in a similar but less aggressive way. The following sentence does not need brackets or even bracketing commas as the "and" is a connective, making commas redundant:

Original student version

This experience got me thinking about how I would react to a patient physically attacking me, whether or whether not the patient had a psychotic condition (and therefore not in complete control of their actions).

Amended version

This experience made me think about how I would react to a patient physically attacking me, whether or not the patient had a psychotic condition and was therefore not in complete control of their actions.

➤ This work also features a classic example of a computer spell-check error. The student relates a doctor speaking in a "clam voice" instead of a calm voice. Whilst a tutor may find this type of mistake amusing for a second, they would probably lose patience with and respect for this student if such errors became commonplace. You must always remember that a computer spellcheck cannot be totally trusted and that careful and objective proofreading is crucial.

Although we follow a number of patients throughout our clinical practice, from start of treatment to when they are discharged, one of the first patients I saw in clinics I followed at the time thinking that it would have no benefit on my education as I never looked at his charts or notes. Instead I built up a rapport with the patient and visited him daily; taking up newspapers and allowing him to talk for sometimes hours about himself and how he was feeling about his wellbeing, his treatment and life in general. Looking back it was probably one of the most educational experiences of my life and although not strictly clinical, lessons learnt are 100% applicable to every patient I encounter from now onwards.

My first encounter with the patient was when an FY1 took us to his room to listen to his heart sounds as he had had a valve replacement and therefore made for an interesting discussion. The patient exchanged his time and exposure for an opportunity to tell us about his experiences as a taxi driver in London and how he took part in a research project on taxi drivers and their memory capacity, which the junior doctor tried to hurry through as there were 8 of us stood around and teaching time was short. Later that day I returned to a patient with a newspaper article I had cut out that was about the research project he had been in which he hadn't seen before and I hung around to explain to him what it all meant.

From then onwards I visited him almost daily and we spoke about everything from the death of his wife to his pride in his grandchildren, and all the cruises in between. However over time I witnessed drastic personality changes in the weeks leading up to his operation as he continued to suffer in pain and felt the surgeons weren't keeping him informed as to what was going on and whether or not they were going to operate on him. He slowly went from eating all of the hospital food provided to eating nothing and eventually being put on an enteral feeding regime, while he drastically lost weight and became more agitated and prone to mood swings. If any medical student had approached him in the later periods he would have become labelled one of the 'difficult patients' and rarely approached again, but from my perspective it was clear the pain and extended confinement in a hospital bed were taking their toll. The surgery was constantly delayed as they tried to bring his weight back up, which was difficult and prolonged, but eventually he was slipped on to an emergency list and prepped for surgery within 48 hours.

In those 48 hours the patient went from angry about delays to scared and not feeling ready to have the operation, not knowing what was going to happen, worried about the colostomy bag he would be left with and fearing his own mortality. I spent significant periods with his in the run up to the operation discussing his fears and reassuring him that the surgeons were acting in his best interests.

Post-operatively I visited him in ITU and he seemed in good spirits, communicating with doctors and looking like his pain was well controlled. It was a relief and naively I assumed from there he was in for a brief recovery on the ward and discharge.

Visiting him again once he had been moved upstairs it was clear that this wasn't the case and his pain was poorly controlled, he looked sicker than I had seen any patients on the ward look and his communication was limited. He started cutting off our conversations after a few minutes and on ward rounds I heard it was almost impossible for the physiotherapists to engage him. While this was worrying enough in itself, I encountered a number of loud arguments between him and nursing staff where he was being aggressive and was genuinely confused, with episodes of paranoia in between. Though I managed to communicate with him during that period, conversations were based around how everyone was out to get him, that the nursing staff were trying to kill him or he was delusional. After a few minutes he would quickly cut off our conversations and ask me to leave. It was extremely upsetting to see such a rapid deterioration in a patient that had been so alert, friendly and responsive and at the time not knowing whether he would recover or not was the most upsetting aspect. I saw his family around on a number of occasions and while previously our conversations had been general and worrying over what he was eating, they were now upset, distressed and always asking about who they could corner to find out what was going on. His bed was directly opposite my locker room and some days I avoided going to it completely as I didn't know what I would say when he engaged with me, although looking back I was selfishly protecting myself from the feelings of helplessness and rejection that plagued me for the entire day after I had been to see him. However, I started to force myself to revisit him and eventually gradual improvements were seen. He started eating again and once he started he didn't stop! On one occasion I trawled Tottenham Court Road to find him a Thai chicken takeaway that he had a craving for but going from seeing a frail old man losing weight by the day to seeing a cheeky smile on his face as he ate from a Wagamamas tub was unbelievable and its impact on me was instantaneous. Although never the same as he was before, not quite as alert or cheeky, he settled down and was prepped for discharge.

The last event in our relationship was the day before he was due to be discharged – I went to visit him to find a distressed and angry man stating that he wanted to kill himself and that his life wasn't worth living any more. I spent the afternoon with him, talking through his fears about going out with a colostomy bag and how no one would notice or be bothered by it, to his concerns about going into a home and his disappointment that his children wouldn't take him in to live with them no matter how much he pleaded. Him going into a home was the issue that hit me the hardest as before the operation he was always talking about how much he couldn't wait to get back into his taxi and get back to work. It was an emotional afternoon but leaving him smiling and chatting to a nurse was the reassurance I needed that I had done the best I could to help him through the emotions he was going through.

In the weeks I spent with the patient playing as much a part of my clinical rotation as my tutorials, I went through all of the patient-doctor relationship moments and emotions I could think of, and more. Looking back on it I hoped I had made an impact on him and helped him through some difficult periods but he impacted on me more than I could have ever impacted on him and he will be a patient I will never forget. It taught me not to judge patients based on how they act towards us, I had let first impressions of patients dominate the way I treated them from then on, failing to take into consideration the variables of pain, distress, malnutrition and fear that impact on the way they behave in hospital. A number of people said at the time that there was no point in me following up the patient this closely as when I was a 'real doctor' I would never have time to build up that kind of relationship with a patient and I have to distance myself from them. My response at the time and would still be, as medical students we are in the privileged position of having time and a lack of actual responsibility for the patients on our side. As FY1s we can rush through patients and try to efficiently manage their care while in the back of our minds running through the millions of other things we need to be doing but as medical students we need to slow down and take time with our patients to learn as much from each of them as possible so the foundations for decent doctor-patient relationships, that are discussed so much in lecture theatres but never at the bedside, are there from the start of our practice. The next three years are the best opportunity we are ever going to get to interact with patients on a personal level and the biggest differences we can make as students is not blood taking or chart fetching, its reaching out to patients that feel neglected, lonely or afraid and being able to use your position to improve their experience.

COMMENTS ON REFLECTION

Although nicely written, this reflective essay is rather disappointing because of the lack of purposeful reflection until the very end. Most of the essay is descriptive. It lacks, for example, a deeper exploration of the author's personal role in events and actions, analytical reflection or the consideration of the judgements and suppositions made and possible alternative explanations.

We are left having to guess whether the author felt that her contact with the patient was helpful to him apart from her hope that she "had made an impact on him and helped him through some difficult periods". The author could have explored what impact she wanted to make and, on reflection, what impact she feels she had made. More thought and detail would be helpful in exploring what way specifically the patient made an impact on her, what will she remember and what she learned.

She also wrote:

A number of people said at the time that there was no point in me following up the patient this closely as when I was a 'real doctor' I would never have time to build up that kind of relationship with a patient and I have to distance myself from them. My response at the time and would still be, as medical students we are in the privileged position of having time and a lack of actual responsibility for the patients on our side.

Does she believe that after qualification doctors do not have the time to establish this sort of relationship with patients?

COMMENTS ON ENGLISH

What was done well

➤ This essay is generally well paragraphed. The student has sensibly divided the essay into a number of different paragraphs that reflect changes in time, subject matter or sentiment. Logical paragraphing aids the fluency of their writing and makes it easier for a reader to follow their thoughts. The only slightly problematic paragraph here is the fourth paragraph, which commences: "Post-operatively I visited him in ITU…" This paragraph is slightly too short (only two sentences long). Paragraphs should be at least three sentences long to justify their independence. When they are too short they can seem undeveloped.

What could have been done better

➤ The main problem with this essay is its syntactical flaws: some sentences are confusingly constructed. Reflective essays are often thematically complex (they deal with complex situations, emotions and outcomes) but they should be grammatically simple and correct. This student has written many confusingly structured sentences that could be simply improved by shortening them or reordering a few words.

Original student version

Although we follow a number of patients throughout our clinical practice, from start of treatment to when they are discharged, one of the first patients I saw in clinics I followed at the time thinking that it would have no benefit on my education as I never looked at his charts or notes.

Amended version

Throughout our clinical course we follow a number of patients from admission to discharge. I initially thought that one of the first patients I met would be of little educational value to me because I had not taken the time to read his notes.

➤ This student also overgeneralises, a poor technique in academic writing. Reflective writing deals with specific situations and reactions and you must ensure that you avoid using broad, sweeping statements as they are often inaccurate and too simplistic.

Original student version

Looking back it was probably one of the most educational experiences of my life and although not strictly clinical, lessons learnt are 100% applicable to every patient I encounter from now onwards.

Amended version

Looking back, it was probably one of the most educational experiences of my student life and, although not strictly clinical, I believe the lessons I learned will be relevant to many patients I will meet.

It was my first 'on take' in the Accident in Emergency department, and one of the junior doctors asked myself and another student to cannulate a patient. The doctor briefly explained that the lady was an alcoholic who had taken an overdose of paracetemol. The patient in question was lying in the bed, curled up and sobbing to herself. I immediately was slightly taken aback and approached the patient. Touching the patient on the shoulder to gain her attention, I introduced myself and asked what the matter was, and if there was anything I could do. The patient sobbed "I want to die; I can't live with what has happened".Upon more questioning, the patient revealed that she had been raped a few days before. She said that she had gone to the police who didn't believe her. My initial reaction was shocked and I felt extremely sorry for the patient; I had never met anyone who had been raped or wanted to commit suicide and couldn't help but imagine the anguish she must be in.

I decided to concentrate at the task at hand, explaining the procedure I had been asked to do, and asking if she understood and if that was ok. The patient continued to cry and eventually said "Do what you want". Taking this as consent, I proceeded to prepare for the cannulation. After cleaning the skin, I warned the patient of a sharp scratch at which she swiftly withdrew her arm. I explained to the patient that the pain would not last long and was necessary for treatment that she might be given. She gave back her arm and allowed the needle to puncture her skin without moving. However, as I was attempting to advance the cannula, the patient started to move her arm to withdraw it, and the arm was also shaking due to her continual sobs. At this point, my colleague had to hold her arm still to allow the cannula to be inserted safely. The patient resisted but I managed to secure the device and explained to the patient to leave it in place. The situation was clearly not ideal both in terms of gaining consent, and in terms of performing the procedure. It was certainly in the patient's best interests to have the cannulation and she had implicitly consented by providing her arm. Whether the patient was in the correct state of mind to understand, weigh up, and retain the information (in order to legally consent to the procedure) was also debatable due to the impact of alcohol and emotional distress. Nonetheless the issue of helping a patient who does not want to be helped was also raised, particularly in the field of mental health and suicide. Furthermore, while the needle was sheathed when the patient jerked away, the importance of universal precautions and general care with sharps was highlighted to me. In hindsight it would have been better to spend more time with the patient, explaining the importance of staying still, and getting her to do so voluntarily.

I sat with the patient for the next hour, taking history but also talking to generally about her life. She lived alone, and had no family, with only one friend. The patient described how she came to be raped, saying the man was someone she worked with who had taken advantage of her while drunk. When the conversation came to an end and the patient was calm, my colleague and excused ourselves. Once out of earshot, the other student suggested to me that her story about the rape may not have been true. I was annoyed that he would make such a judgement about her, assuming that because she was an alcoholic she could not be trusted. The comment re- emphasised to me that as medical professionals our job is not to make value judgements on a patient's lifestyle or to make assumptions about their morals. Certainly it is practically necessary in most situations to take what a patient says as truth. However, while this is true, it is important to be aware that patients may have their own agendas, for example in drug or attention seeking behaviour. It is also possible to recognise that certain groups of people are more likely to have other issues (medical and non medical) without judging or discriminating against those groups-for example, alcoholics are more likely to have psychiatric disorders. Alcoholism can indeed be seen as a medical addiction. Moreover, I learnt that the impact of psychosocial factors in medical problems cannot be underestimated. In this case, the patient's lack of a social support network and apparent deficit of social interaction was perhaps both a cause and a perpetuating factor in her alcoholism and were hindering how she dealt with the rape. To this end, it perhaps is not always sufficient to treat the presenting medical problem, in this case, overdose, but also the multiple problems associated with it, such as depression, alcoholism, and social factors.

COMMENTS ON REFLECTION

This is a second piece by the same author as the last essay and the development of her reflective writing is evident. Apart from one missed opportunity to reflect further and try to make some sense of the situation when she writes about stereotyping and its uses, this is a lovely piece. It is a delight for a reflective practice tutor to see this sort of development in reflection and reflective writing after giving careful feedback.

COMMENTS ON ENGLISH
What was done well
➤ The overall quality of the English here is impressive. The student has used paragraphs well, structured sentences sensibly and used a range of vocabulary, which all makes for accurate and precise writing and, therefore, enjoyable reading.

What could have been done better
➤ Whilst the general quality of the written English is good, there are a few unnecessary commas here. Commas are used to indicate where your reader should pause and, whilst you do not want them to be out of breath when reading your work, too many unnecessary stops can actually confuse the meaning of your work. The following sentences include four commas yet the only necessary comma is the one following the word "however". All of the other commas should be removed:

However, as I was attempting to advance the cannula, the patient started to move her arm to withdraw it, and the arm was also shaking due to her continual sobs. At this point, my colleague had to hold her arm still to allow the cannula to be inserted safely. The patient resisted but I managed to secure the device and explained to the patient to leave it in place. The situation was clearly not ideal both in terms of gaining consent, and in terms of performing the procedure.

When beginning this project, the task seemed fairly simple; to learn about cancer by focussing on the case history of one patient. However, upon further consideration, the task becomes more complex when deciding whether the main is to gain experience on the medical, scientific dimension of cancers or on the human, emotional one. It became clear, as time went on the two aspects are not entirely separate, and that a full scientific understanding of cancer and its multifaceted effects on the patient, requires engagement on a personal level.

Of course, this was never simple, and my first meeting SM, a 69 year old Cypriot male, was during his first round of chemotherapy. The initial history taking seemed fairly simple, as SM had a clear history and was initially quite talkative considering the situation. However, when I asked about his feelings, it seemed to trigger an internal recoiling within him. He became quite defensive, and seemed to underplay the effect his diagnosis had on him, commenting that his generation of men did not moan about their illnesses. I immediately realised the importance of building a strong rapport with the patient before approaching certain subjects, and indeed the effect that the patients age, gender and culture has on their approach to their own feelings. It also became clear what kind of questions patients may expect from medical professionals, as strikingly, SM had been happy to talk in detail about his bowel habit, but did not want to admit any feelings of shock or sadness upon his diagnosis.

After this first encounter with SM, we met several more times. I became better at talking to him about his feelings, mainly by asking indirect and open questions to give him the opportunity to answer them how he liked. He shared with me that he had been feeling depressed and socially isolated following the end of his chemoradiotherapy. He commented on how he thought this had accentuated and worsened his apparent symptoms of pain. I also met his son, which had mixed effects. Firstly I was able to develop a real sense of SM's family life, and also gage the effects on his family, as the son was much more forthcoming about his feelings of fear and anger. However, as SM's son was approximately my age, the generational gap between me and SM was highlighted. Moreover, on a personal level, I found myself confronting my own family's mortality. My last meeting with SM and his son was an extremely positive one, with encouraging MRI results, and a massive turnaround in SM's mood. He seemed to be feeling much better and for the first time I heard him speak of looking forward to something; the summer. I was really pleased to hear of SM's improvement, although all too aware that the outcome for a different patient may not have been so.

COMMENTS ON REFLECTION

An encounter with a patient who had a profound effect on you is a good episode to reflect upon. Often, patients shape a doctor's attitudes and clinical behaviour, and here the author exposes a change from seeing someone as a patient to someone who is a whole person with a life and a family as well as an illness. The piece is a bit short and could do with another paragraph or two of critical reflection exploring the learning and professional growth that has come from the obviously very meaningful encounter.

In the third paragraph there is an unfortunate choice of wording. The author describes the "apparent symptoms" as if they were fictitious or over-egged. It is clear this is not what the author meant but it causes some doubt for the reader.

COMMENTS ON ENGLISH
What was done well

➤ This essay is well paragraphed. The student has clearly divided her essay into an introduction that introduces and outlines the nature of the incident, a second paragraph that describes the incident and a third paragraph that develops the incident and its effects on the student. Designing a logically planned and structured essay is important and if you are in doubt about how to do so refer to Figure 2.1.

What could have been done better

➤ This essay features some very confusing sentences and grammatical glitches that could have been ironed out by some proofreading alone or with a peer. Reflective writing usually deals with a complex situation or complex emotional reactions that must be communicated in accurate sentences or else meaning is warped; the opening paragraph here is particularly unclear. Many students use their opening paragraph as a "warm-up" paragraph and as a result end up with grammatically mangled introductions. Your introduction should be one of the strongest parts of your essay and it is worth spending time perfecting it as it introduces and justifies your choice of topic. This student has obviously rushed her introduction, which could be simply improved by reordering, refining and shortening some sentences and ensuring that tenses agree, to improve clarity:

Original student version

When beginning this project, the task seemed fairly simple; to learn about cancer by focussing on the case history of one patient. However, upon further consideration, the task becomes more complex when deciding whether the main is to gain experience on the medical, scientific dimension of cancers or on the human, emotional one. It became clear, as time went on the two aspects are not entirely separate, and that a full scientific understanding of cancer and its multifaceted effects on the patient, requires engagement on a personal level.

Amended version

My initial thought about this project was to learn about cancer using a patient's case history. I was unsure whether I should focus on the medical and scientific aspects of cancers or on the human and emotional aspects. I then decided that all these topics were important components of the project, because a comprehensive understanding of cancer and its multifaceted effects on the patient requires personal interaction between the doctor and patient.

I have decided to reflect on a recent experience of what I perceived to be poor teaching style. This occurred after a student had presented a clerking to one of the consultants. The clerking that he had presented did not follow the exact format that the consultant had wanted us to follow, nevertheless it was thorough apart from a few minor errors that any one of the group could have made. Once the student had finished, the consultant proceeded to say that he considered it to be one of the worst clerkings he had heard in the last five years, it was surprising for someone who appeared so bright to perform so poorly, and that he was shocked that the student had not been spoken to earlier. His criticism and manner in my opinion was far from constructive and was in fact quite rude, yet the student decided to remain quiet and not defend himself.

My initial reaction was that this was a simple case of teaching through humiliation. As time has gone by, we have all developed a thick skin and learned to not be too disheartened by the words of one consultant, and the student was reacting how many of us would, by keeping quiet. However in this case, the consultant's words were more than just humiliation. He was belittling, rude, and they were the kind of comments that could have made a less self-assured medical student think twice about whether they were in the right career. I wondered how I would feel had I been placed in my fellow student's position; I am quite sure that I would have been much more obviously upset. I felt embarrassed for my colleague, and uncomfortable for him, not to mention shocked and angry at the consultant for making a fellow student feel so inadequate, when he clearly was not. Following the encounter, I thought that the student had come off the as the more mature, and also realised the importance of having other consultants that are more constructive with criticism, and understanding of the fact that we do not know as much as they do; thereby helping to maintain a positive, and importantly, enjoyable working environment for the students.

One of the key positive aspects that I took from the experience were that I realised it is important to use your firm as a support network, as following the event, which the entire firm had witnessed, we were all as supportive as possible towards the medical student, which was extremely important as he felt very isolated and singled out. It also strengthened my belief in the fact that there is no excuse for rudeness and that although some consultants believe that it is ok to act in this way towards students, it is most certainly not, and as a result, it is important to not allow this type of consultant crush your confidence in yourself. A final positive point in my opinion was the student's reaction, or rather, non reaction to the consultant's words. There is alot that he may have fairly said back to the consultant, but he remained diplomatic and although some may have seen this as weak, I think that it was particularly strong and difficult to do this. The obvious negative aspect of the event was the manner in which the consultant gave his criticism. I feel as though his tone of voice and the selection of words could have been much more tactful, and he could have made the same point in a less destructive way. It is surprising that a person who had been teaching for so long would adopt this approach towards teaching, and that he was allowed to get away with his behaviour, but evidently, he is probably not the only consultant who has acted this way, and I wonder if he was also taught in the same way.

On further analysis, I can see that the consultant probably did not mean to come across so negatively and he was trying to help, and perhaps this is the only way that he could ensure that his points would be remembered. It is true that the experience will not be forgotten, but it is for reasons that are likely different to the object of the tutorial, to remember a Case to aid our memory. However, I can see that a consultant with years of experience behind him, having most staff follow his instructions would be irritated by students who do not follow his instructions exactly, as is likely the case during his normal working day. This is likely to be why his irritation was so obvious. It is also quite likely that he, like many consultants would not be used to having other people tell him that the way he has acted may be inappropriate and I feel that if this had not been the case, he may have been more tactful in his approach.

I can conclude that my experience of 'the rude consultant' is one that is not essential but extremely useful for medical students during the course of their training. It shows the importance of being a good teacher to future students, giving them motivation to become better doctors in a constructive and not destructive way. It also taught me that the firm is an important source of support during the difficult and upsetting times that everyone experiences during the medical course.

In the future, I will endeavour to be as supportive as possible to medical students that I may teach, and remember the impact of having a good teacher and role model. As a medical student I will continue to remember that I am more than comfortable with my decision to be a doctor, and that a single negative experience should not erase this.

COMMENTS ON REFLECTION

This is a satisfactory reflective piece. The author has unpicked the emotional responses of both herself and the other student in the incident and described her discomfort about the consultant's teaching style, empathising with the student who she feels was humiliated. There is a thin line between teaching directly and a student's perception of humiliation, which could be partly embarrassment about a poor-quality presentation. The author mentions that the consultant had already laid down the ground rules for the way he liked students to present and so there may have been some justification for his criticism of the student.

The author describes reflection-in-action: her own emotions of shock, embarrassment and discomfort with the way the consultant spoke to the other student and her admiration of the response of the other student. The author then moves on to reflection-on-action: exploring motives and alternative explanations, trying to put herself in her fellow student's shoes and also trying to see the event from the consultant's perspective, looking for possible positive aspects of the consultant's criticism.

She has reflected and learned from the incident. The author concludes that the experience was helpful in showing students how not to teach, and that she will teach in a positive way to motivate students. She does not, unfortunately, provide any details or information about how she would do this or deal with a similar scenario if she were the teacher. The essay is therefore incomplete and the reader is not told what practical teaching message she learned other than her view that she would not teach like "the rude consultant". A good reflective piece provides the reader with a message that they too could learn from.

COMMENTS ON ENGLISH

What was done well

➤ This student has used a good range of appropriate vocabulary that allows the reader to easily follow and relate to the incident. Selecting a range of interesting vocabulary is important when describing a series of complex events and emotions; succinct and precise expression is key. Here is an extract that is particularly strong for these reasons:

He was belittling, rude, and they were the kind of comments that could have made a less self-assured medical student think twice about whether they were in the right career. I wondered how I would feel had I been placed in my fellow student's position; I am quite sure that I would have been much more obviously upset. I felt embarrassed for my colleague, and uncomfortable for him, not to mention shocked and angry at the consultant for making a fellow student feel so inadequate, when he clearly was not.

What could have been done better

➤ Whilst most of this essay is well written, certain sentences are too long and "overstuffed". Reflective writing demands precise expression, as the situations recounted can be complex enough without complicated phrasing. Short sentences are usually always clearer than long sentences. The following extract could be improved by dividing the long sentences into shorter ones as this improves the clarity and pace of the work:

Original student version

The clerking that he had presented did not follow the exact format that the consultant had wanted us to follow, nevertheless it was thorough apart from a few minor errors that any one of the group could have made. Once the student had finished, the consultant proceeded to say that he considered it to be one of the worst clerkings he had heard in the last five years, it was surprising for someone who appeared so bright to perform so poorly, and that he was shocked that the student had not been spoken to earlier. His criticism and manner in my opinion was far from constructive and was in fact quite rude, yet the student decided to remain quiet and not defend himself.

Amended version

The clerking that he had presented did not follow the exact format that the consultant had wanted us to follow. Nevertheless, it was thorough, apart from a few minor errors that any one of the group could have made. Once the student had finished, the consultant said that he considered it to be one of the worst clerkings he had heard in the last five years. He said he found it surprising for someone who appeared so bright to perform so poorly and that he was shocked that the student had not been spoken to earlier. His criticism and manner in my opinion were far from constructive and he was quite rude. However, the student decided to remain quiet and not defend himself.

➤ When proofreading your work it is important to check that all nouns and verbs "agree": singular nouns must be followed by a singular verb and plural nouns by plural verbs. The student has confused their plurals and singulars here as they recount "one of the key aspects", which is obviously singular, yet they used the plural verb "were" instead of "was". Whilst this type of error may seem relatively minor, it looks incredibly sloppy and indicates a lack of careful proofreading.

Original student version
One of the key positive aspects that I took from the experience were that I realised it is important to use your firm as a support network . . .

Amended version
One of the key positive aspects that I took from the experience was that I realised it is important to use your firm as a support network . . .

On clerking a patient admitted to the Acute Admissions Unit at UCH, I was closing the session and found that I was feeling very pleased; I had obtained a very thorough and detailed history that I felt had flowed nicely. An integral part of the satisfaction I had felt with this clerking was due to the fact that I had developed a good rapport with the patient, and she really seemed to open up to me and feel comfortable with talking to me. I thanked the lady and was about to leave when she said: I have some questions for you; "What's ascites and who gets ascites"? I was rather taken aback and was perplexed as to why she was asking me, so asked her directly for the reason behind this enquiry. "I heard the doctors discuss amongst themselves when they came to see me that I had ascites, but they didn't say anything to me so I just left it. They mentioned a few other words too but I can't remember what now." This made me feel distinctly uncomfortable as I knew that the lady was still undergoing investigations, and had not yet been diagnosed. I felt nervous and worried; I did not want to slip up and say something that would cause further anxiousness on the patient's part or get me into trouble with the doctors. We had been taught on several occasions about what to do if you find yourself in such a situation with a patient, however, put on the spot I suddenly could not think of what to say or do. Should I tell her what ascites meant, seeing as I did know but not go into the differential diagnoses as it may cause further concern and worry for the patient? No, I should just go and find a doctor to address the issues raised by the patient. I told the lady that seeing as I was not able to help her, I would go and find a doctor to talk to her, however, she insisted that she did not want to see the doctor and that she would probably see one later on in the day anyway. To my surprise, I actually felt quite relieved, as I myself felt quite apprehensive about approaching the doctors. Having only been on the wards for a few weeks I felt quite intimidated by the busy doctors, but surely my concern for the patient should have overridden any nervousness or lack of confidence on my part with regards to talking to a doctor? At this point I wished the patient all the best and walked away.

It was amazing how satisfied I had felt during the course of the main body of the clerking, but after the patient asking me two seemingly simple questions, I now felt distinctly unsatisfied and disappointed in myself. Even though I had obtained a really good history regarding the patient's presenting complaint, I had not addressed another important aspect of the clerking; the issue of a patient's ideas, concerns and expectations. The patient had felt comfortable enough to express a worry to me; a concern that needed to be and should have been clarified, and in return I had done nothing to help her. I left her in the same situation that she had been in when I first arrived to see her: in the dark. I was deeply disappointed in myself for not handling the situation in a better way. The patient had been of benefit to me in my medical training, but I had been of no use to her. This experience highlighted an important realisation; that my role as a medical student on the wards is one of responsibility too, and I also have a duty of care to the patients. Even if I did not have the answers to the patient's questions, I should have done my utmost to address a very specific issue raised by her.

Looking back at the situation, I think I should have gone to talk to the doctor in charge and explained everything that had happened, as well as the fact that the patient had not wanted me to consult the doctor. Although the wishes of a patient should always be respected, I think it is important for those involved in the patient's care to be aware of such a worry so as to act in the patient's best interests, and help alleviate any distress.

Beyond my own conduct, it then also occurred to me that good communication between the patient and her doctors had also been lacking. The doctors should not have discussed the patient amongst themselves without also feeding back to the patient. Medical terms should not have been used without clarification in the patient's presence, and if the doctors did not want to discuss the patient's condition with her at that point they should have gone into a private room. Such a distance between the patients and doctors and a lack of communication had created a situation in which the patient felt unable to talk to the doctors. Good communication is such a vital part of the patient-doctor partnership, and the patient must have felt extremely uneasy being discussed as though she was not there and hearing conditions that she did not know the meaning or severity of, that she apparently had.

Both a student and doctor have a responsibility to prioritise the care and needs of a patient. It thus follows that in a similar situation, I hope that I will no longer let my own qualms or lack of confidence get in the way of helping a patient. It is also important to remember that as a doctor, it is imperative not just to treat the condition from which the patient is suffering, but also to remember the psychosocial element involved in any patient interaction and to practice good communication.

COMMENTS ON REFLECTION

This is a good reflective piece, written in the first person, with practically all the necessary ingredients. The patient's direct and fair question left the author feeling uncomfortable and disappointed with himself for several reasons. This sort of situation, where things are not properly sorted, leaving uncomfortable feelings about a patient encounter, provides a powerful focus for reflection, allowing professionals to think carefully about what they felt and learned from the encounter. This is a difficult scenario for medical students and the author's reflection shows real professional growth.

The author unfairly denigrates himself: "I had been of no use to her". Had he asked her, she would probably have contradicted him because of his sensitivity, professional and caring response, the time he spent with her and the way he listened to and spoke with her. She would have sensed that he wanted to help her. The consultation in medicine is often very therapeutic.

The author also reflected on bedside discussion between doctors. Whilst he quite rightly does not condone the practice of debate around the bedside, which if not done correctly can unsettle and worry patients, he misses the opportunity to explore why this sort of incident happens.

COMMENTS ON ENGLISH
What was done well
➤ This essay is generally well written, the sentences are sensibly constructed, the

punctuation is appropriate and the work is well ordered and effectively worded. The following extract is particularly strong and exemplifies the aforementioned attributes as well as a good variety of sentence constructions:

Should I tell her what ascites meant, seeing as I did know but not go into the differential diagnoses as it may cause further concern and worry for the patient? No, I should just go and find a doctor to address the issues raised by the patient. I told the lady that seeing as I was not able to help her, I would go and find a doctor to talk to her, however, she insisted that she did not want to see the doctor and that she would probably see one later on in the day anyway.

If you are concerned that your essay sounds dull, try experimenting by including in your essay rhetorical questions, long descriptive sentences, and short emphatic sentences. This mix makes the essay varied, more interesting and enjoyable to read and write.

➤ The student has also used an effective range of vocabulary to capture the emotions and situations recounted. Words such as "amazing", "relieved", "surprised" and "intimidated" are all vivid and clear. Sometimes the best descriptions are the lightest on words and yet still deliver maximum impact. Reflective writing is a deeply personal exercise and flowery writing can often frustrate, not elucidate, your account.

What could have been done better
This essay is mostly very good and there are not many holes in its composition or effect.

"Mrs AB came to the hospital on the 12th of September, she presented with shortness of breath, nausea and chest pain..."

"Right, give me three differentials" said Dr E, the Consultant.

My firm turned as one and looked at me, their eyes saying exactly what I'd be thinking in their place: thank God it's not me. I began to sweat, my mouth went dry, and I shuffled my notes thinking surely my palpitations must be audible right across the ward. I tried to coax my brain into producing a coherent sound, preferably a medical one, and as the words formed, a fellow student interjected with "could it be gastroenteritis sir".

There was silence around the bed, Mrs AB sat up and looked at the student (let us call him Bill) who looked at us and we in turn looked at Dr E, who was not happy.

"Three years at UCL, phase 1 and an intercalated BSc. have taught you that gastroenteritis is the first differential to S.O.B, chest pain and nausea in a 68 year old overweight lady! What is the first differential does anybody know?" Dr E exclaimed.

At that point we were all in a state of complete academic panic; one member of my firm rifled through the oxford handbook madly, the other clutched the baby Kumar and Clark with fervent adoration and a third mounted a covert operation toward the notes at the foot of Mrs AB's bed. Reviewing the situation now, at the end of my first rotation, the presentation of a first differential is not so daunting. However in September it was another matter completely. Our knowledge base was wide and scattered throughout many different fields. We could tell you odd facts about adenosine receptors, or the sequencing of HLA genes and I personally, can recite the Medicines Sans Frontiers 12 priorities but somehow could not think about what Mrs AB's diagnosis was. The last week of pathology teaching was a blur of lectures and time spent trying to stay awake whilst making reams of notes in awful handwriting. Although at least now we know what a differential diagnosis actually means. In the first week a student dared to ask in a tutorial what a doctor meant when discussing differentials, suffice to say that it did not end well.

Let us return to the presentation at hand.

Dr E was still waiting, his face is flicked from one student to the next measuring our ability to provide him with valid answers. Somehow I don't think he was impressed so far and his estimation in our firm was falling rapidly with each passing moment. Finally another student provided him with "myocardial infarction" and we all could breathe. Thus began my first day on the wards as a clinical student and I felt wholly inadequate.

Pre-clinical medicine taught us the science, the essential details and principles that are core to understanding the disease processes occurring in the patients we see. Clinical medicine aims to bring that to a higher context, place our (supposed) knowledge and give it literal flesh. Growing up around family who are mostly doctors had already given me an insight into the realities of medical life but I was still overwhelmed by the experience of entering phase 2. The university does its best at preparing us, the lectures, the handouts and countless pastel coloured guides. However, only the act of being in clinics teaches you both the best and worst aspects of medicine. I believe that this aspect of the course is wholly underestimated: the power of clinical medicine to completely re-shape the identity of what medicine as a course means to a student. We all enter medicine with varying degrees of certainty, some of us know where we are headed (or like to think so), whilst others simply are in it for the experience. We all laud our predecessors, masters in the age old vocation of medicine. However in truth when it comes to it, clinical teaching shines the unforgiving light of reality onto our dreams, which many find difficult to resolve. The things which we were most excited about may turn out to be something we actually hate. For me the most exciting part was the prospect of being in a hospital, watching live surgery, reading x-rays and taking blood, real doctor stuff. What I've found to be the most fulfilling aspect is all that hands on experience and more especially the time we get to work with the patients and doctors in the hospital.

I am amazed daily by the expertise, knowledge and complete professionalism displayed by the staff. Doctors, nurses, physiotherapists, health care workers all dancing around the patient, running from ward to ward and still managing to drag us along for teaching. This is the real world of medicine that I signed up for. Of course there are bad days, days where sessions are cancelled, days where Dr E asks really difficult questions and where staff and students are rude. On a cold, wet and dark winter morning not all of us are wholeheartedly excited to go into diabetic outpatient clinic and look at feet for four hours. Surprisingly it has been such times when I have learned the most from my teachers, the times when I have seen patient after patient with the same condition so repetitively that there is no way I'm going to forget about the signs of diabetes. It is easy at this stage in our career to become arrogant, confident and dismissive of the so called softer specialities and though we are diffident around the wards collectively we can completely overwrite certain aspects of medicine.

The sword of temperance to this fate is our abject lack of knowledge. Eleven weeks into our rotation we may know how to examine the major systems and take a functional history of the knee. The diligent among us even know how to interpret ECGs and present in trauma meetings but there will always be a Dr E with just that one question we will never know the answer to. Although this is frustrating and the mountain of learning seemingly insurmountable this is in fact the cornerstone of our development in this chosen vocation of ours. To be challenged, probed and found wanting is the most vital driving force we have; for medicine is nothing if not a profession of curiosity and the constant endeavour to know, excel and continue to learn.

Bill clerked a patient with supposedly no previous hospital admissions and on presenting to the infamous Dr E was confident that this time there was no aspect of the case he wasn't completely sure of, but medicine still has a way of surprising you, the thing I've found is that we can't let go of our sense of humour:
"So you picked up on his bilateral leg amputation right? Talk me through the management plan for Mr R" grinned Dr E,
poor Bill.

COMMENTS ON REFLECTION

This piece has an engaging start that brings the reader right into the moment. This is a useful device for reflective writing, but not enough. The essay is quite well written and has some amusing bits for the casual reader, but is rather immature. It does not contain enough personal reflection for a serious piece and is therefore unsatisfactory, and this is the reason we have included it. Humour and creativity are welcome in reflective writing but without serious reflection they are insufficient.

The use of the word "we" instead of "I" and the references to "Bill" leave the reader with the impression that this is simply an attempt to joke about his colleague's experience on a ward round.

The introduction to a reflective piece should be a brief description of the situation or setting, transporting the reader to where you were and what you were doing. The first 200 words of this essay are superfluous and could be replaced by a sentence or two stating that the scene was a consultant bedside teaching round held in the first few weeks of his clinical course. This highlights the importance of understanding what reflection is and why, as a learner, you are being asked to write reflectively. Writing the essay, saving it and then rereading it after a day or two (this necessitates adequate preparation time) with a critical objective eye will often highlight that you have missed the point. It might also have encouraged this author to keep the sentences pertinent and simple, check the spelling, punctuation and grammar, keep to the required word count and so forth.

COMMENTS ON ENGLISH

What was done well

➤ The conversational style in which the student has chosen to write their essay is engaging and interesting to read. Although writing direct speech (directly spoken dialogue that appears in speech marks) is often tricky to get right, this student has succeeded in making their writing logical and interesting, and the opening, in particular, is very effective.

➤ The student has used some ambitious and descriptive vocabulary, which also enlivens their account. Whilst your reflective essay should not sound like a poem, do attempt to vary and develop your language. The student uses words such as "rapidly", "diligent" and "abject", making their writing sound more sophisticated. However, remember to use words appropriately and if you have any doubts about what they mean, particularly if English is not your first language, ask someone else who is good at English to check your work and the vocabulary.

What could have been done better

➤ This essay is disappointing grammatically because of some careless punctuation errors. When writing a question, whether in direct speech or a rhetorical question, you must end the sentence with a question mark instead of a full stop:

Original student version

. . . "could it be gastroenteritis sir".

Amended version

. . . "could it be gastroenteritis, Sir?"

➤ The student has also neglected to capitalise the first letters of some proper nouns: *Oxford Handbook* should begin with a capital letter. *See* Chapter 2 for more information regarding the correct use of capital letters.

One incident that really stands out in my mind occurred while on-take in Accident and Emergency. I had been on-take since 8.00PM, and it seemed that we were experiencing an unusually quiet night in A&E. A few patients had already been seen to and clerked and were now asleep and there was no one in the waiting room. At about 2.00AM, there was finally some activity when a middle-aged man was brought into A&E by the paramedics, who hadn't managed to get any information from the man regarding his details or his reasons for coming into hospital. The registrar on-take then approached the man, and spent a significant number of minutes trying to find out the patients name. It soon became clear, after a few slurred words that the man was inebriated, and this seemed to anger the registrar to a great extent, and his manner became very aggressive. He proceeded to shout angrily at the patient and questioned him as to why he had come in to A&E. 'I've hurt my back,' the man replied, to which the doctor responded: 'Then go home and take some painkillers. You don't come into the hospital for that. Have you lost all sense of what is appropriate? This behaviour is not appropriate!' The doctor's tirade at the patient continued for about 10 minutes, while the doctor shouted rudely and loudly at the patient and everyone else in the ward simply looked on or ignored what was happening.

I sat quietly and did not address the situation, even after the man had been sent away and the doctor had returned to his post next to us, but the whole scenario had affected me considerably. I began to think about the manner in which the doctor had behaved and questioned weather this had really been the best course of action. After all, I could understand his frustration at a patient who had come into the hospital, clearly drunk and who had then behaved in an uncooperative manner. Had this been a particularly busy night on A&E, this behaviour would have been even more exasperating. No one else on-take seemed to have been at all surprised or flustered by the incident and this made me believe that this may have been a regular occurrence. The nurse confirmed that this was true – many people came into A&E for no reason other than inebriation. I tried to understand the doctor's position – this was not a solitary episode, and it must be both trying and infuriating to deal with such patients on a regular basis. On top of this, the doctor had wasted time that could have been better spent simply trying to get the patient to respond to him.

However, I still felt uncomfortable with the whole scenario. I could not help but feel that the doctor had been excessively rude and aggressive towards the patient. After all, the man had come into A&E and, despite the fact that he was drunk he deserved to be treated with respect, as all other patients do. I felt that the doctor had not acted in accordance with the guidelines set out by the GMC. These clearly state that a doctor must treat patients as individuals and respect their dignity and to treat patients politely and considerately. The doctor had undoubtedly not acted correspondingly. In addition, the GMC guidelines state that a doctor should be open and honest and act with integrity, ensuring that they do not discriminate unfairly against patients nor abuse their patients trust in them. In my belief, the doctor had done both – he had immediately judged the patient for being under the influence of alcohol and had therefore proceeded to discriminate against him. He had not allowed for the fact, that despite the patient being drunk, he may have had a viable medical complaint that needed seeing to and that perhaps the patient was in need of hospital care. The doctor had also abused the trust that the patient placed in him and the medical profession to offer medical care – perhaps the next time this man finds himself needing to visit A&E, he will think twice after remembering the anger of the doctor. In my opinion the doctor had behaved both unsuitably and unprofessionally.

I then attempted to put myself in the doctor's position. How would I have reacted if I had been in the same situation? After all, I am sure it is difficult to show kindness and compassion to a patient who turns up in A&E intoxicated at 2.00AM in the morning. The doctor did make some valid points to the patient – the behaviour of the patient was inappropriate and perhaps it was necessary to convey this to him. But, had I been the doctor on-take I would like to think I would broach the subject in a different manner and calmly explain to the patient that his behaviour was not acceptable and point out that time-wasting was dangerous and unfair to other patients. I would listen to the patient's complaint properly, and try to find out more about it, rather than dismiss it as this particular doctor had done as this could be detrimental to the patients well-being.

Overall, the incident made me think about the manner in which a doctor should conduct him or herself. What I witnessed that night made me think more seriously about the type of doctor I wish to be in the future. While I understand that it can be easy to get angry and frustrated in situations such as this one, I don't believe it is right to take this anger out on the patients. The behaviour of the patient was wrong, but in my opinion, so was the doctor's. In addition, it also provided me with a real insight into being a doctor in A&E – and the fact that dealing with intoxicated patients is a reality and something that I will probably have to face fairly regularly.

At the time, I didn't mention the incident to the doctor and I didn't attempt to raise the topic with him, feeling that as a medical student it would be presumptuous to tell the registrar that I was uncomfortable with his behaviour. In retrospect, I suppose I could have questioned the doctor about his reaction to better understand why he had acted so abrasively and perhaps let him know that I felt he had been too harsh on the patient. The next time an incident such as this occurs, I might feel more inclined to let my feelings be known. However, I believe that for me the scenario was important because it made me think. Experiences such as this, and reflection upon them are beneficial in making me think seriously and honestly about my future behaviour as a doctor. Sometimes when you view a situation objectively you can see it more clearly and therefore when I do qualify as a doctor I will try to remember that I should attempt to view myself from the patient's perspective. Hopefully, this will ensure that I always treat my patients with respect, and maintain their dignity.

COMMENTS ON REFLECTION

This is a good piece of reflection. The reader is left in no doubt about the situation and can easily visualise the scene in the Accident and Emergency cubicle. The author is quite perceptive and correct in his assessment of both the patient and the behaviour of the doctor. He has intelligently put himself in the position of both and reflected on what he saw, what he felt, what he did and did not do (discuss his feelings with the registrar) and what he learned from the experience.

COMMENTS ON ENGLISH

What was done well

➤ This essay is well structured and paragraphed. Each paragraph deals with a slightly different part of the story or reflection and thus the sequence of events is easy for the reader to follow.

➤ The student uses a rhetorical question to further reflection: "I then attempted to put myself in the doctor's position. How would I have reacted if I had been in the same situation?" Rhetorical questions (questions that provoke thoughts rather than demand answers) are an effective way of varying sentence structure and pace in reflective essays. A few more questions engage the reader's interest and emphasise that the essay is reflective. The sentence could be improved by deleting "if" to read 'How would I have reacted had I been in the same situation'.

What could have been done better

➤ The student includes some direct speech in the opening paragraph. Direct speech is where the actual speech is reported in speech marks. Indirect speech is usually more appropriate in pieces of formal academic writing.

Original student version

He proceeded to shout angrily at the patient and questioned him as to why he had come in to A&E. 'I've hurt my back,' the man replied, to which the doctor responded: 'Then go home and take some painkillers. You don't come into the hospital for that. Have you lost all sense of what is appropriate? This behaviour is not appropriate!'

Amended version

He proceeded to shout angrily at the patient and questioned him as to why he had come into A&E. The man claimed he had hurt his back. The doctor responded in an angry and frustrated way, telling the patient to go home and take some painkillers, reprimanding him for his inappropriate behaviour.

➤ The student uses dashes a lot. Whilst you may see them in media texts, dashes are rarely appropriate in formal academic writing. Usually full stops, commas, colons or semicolons are better substitutes. Remember that words after a semicolon do have to be grammatically complete whereas a colon can be followed by a "non-sentence":

Original student version

The doctor did make some valid points to the patient – the behaviour of the patient was inappropriate and perhaps it was necessary to convey this to him.

Amended version

The doctor did make some valid points to the patient; the behaviour of the patient was inappropriate and perhaps it was necessary to convey this to him.

On Acute Admission Unit (AAU) at UCLH I spent Saturday 14th of November on take and clerked a 79 year old lady who had presented with loss of consciousness. As I started to clerk the patient, I soon realised it was not going to be a quick exercise. The lady had left her glasses and hearing aid at home, and as a result every question had to be broken down, keeping my mouth close to her ear so she had the best chance of hearing my questions. Often my questions had to be repeated and rephrased. As the clerking progressed I learnt that she had emigrated from East Germany, had never married, lived alone, and had a history of depression. I also found out that she had actually lost consciousness whilst collecting free newspapers to take back to her immobile and infirm neighbours. Several times I found my self becoming frustrated with sluggish pace of the interview, well aware that my Saturday evening was being consumed. However, I pushed these thoughts aside, realising that here was an isolated, fragile lady who had come to harm trying to do good for other people. The least that I could do was take my time and listen to her story. Roughly two hours later I had finished clerking the patient and headed home.

During the following week the patient was kept on AAU for monitoring. Every time I passed her, she was sat staring into space, and never had any visitors with her. On most occasions I would say a brief hello, and if had a few minutes, ask how she was doing. Over the course of the week she appeared to be improving, remarking that she was getting her strength back, and that she was really looking forward to going home. With each meeting I felt a growing rapport and friendship with the patient. On one occasion she attracted my attention as I passed her on the ward, and asked me to ring her neighbour who was expecting her home, as the doctors had delayed her discharge by an extra day. This highlighted to me, that perhaps the nurses and doctors were not paying her enough attention, as one would have expected her to at least be able to ask the nurse this request. The patient did admit to being someone who did not like to cause trouble or bother. Even so, it did feel at times that perhaps the staff took advantage of the fact that she was isolated and had difficulty communicating. The next Wednesday, I was on AAU checking another patients details on CDR. I noticed that in the list of patients I had checked recently, her name was highlighted in black. What did this mean? Had she been discharged? I scanned my eyes to the bottom on the screen, and found the legend. Black = Deceased. She had passed away two days earlier; this was the first patient I knew who had passed away.

My initial reaction was one of subdued shock at the sudden, unexplained death of the patient. The shock was muted perhaps by the additional feeling of confusion over what emotions I was feeling, and indeed which emotions I thought I should have been feeling. As one might expect with a patient I had formed a relationship and strong rapport with, there was a component of sadness. I also felt a sense of guilt for several reasons: guilt at the fact that I had not seen her closer to the time of her death; guilt that I had not found out about her death earlier/checked her progress more recently; guilt that perhaps I had not picked up on some symptoms or signs that may have alerted medics to her imminent deterioration; guilt that I was not more upset. I also felt a sense of injustice, grounded perhaps in my belief that the team were not paying enough attention to the needs of the patient; that some how they could have prevented her death had they been more aware of her. After some consideration I began to realise that perhaps her death was inevitable, and that there was nothing that I or any one else could have done. This sense of helplessness was followed by a sobering awareness that this is probably the first of many such events in my career as a doctor. Finally on top of these largely negative emotions, I began to feel a sense of self satisfaction that I had fulfilled my role as a medical student and provided companionship to a lonely lady in the final days of her life.

Overall I believe that the reaction was natural and nothing to be particularly concerned about. Medical students will obviously all respond differently the first time a patient whom they have built a relationship with dies. The way I responded may have been different according to the circumstances of the patient's death. It bothered me initially that there was no definitive response to the patient's death. It now feels that I needed to have my first experience of a patient's death to act as a yardstick; the initial measurement on a scale of emotion and reaction, to which I will compare similar future events. Only when I have had more experience in dealing in the death of a patient, will I begin notice trends in my emotional responses. Therefore it would seem I am playing a rather morbid waiting game, anticipating where the next measurement will fall on my scale. The experience of the first death of a patient, along with this reflective activity, has taught me the value of reviewing the reactive and emotional content of my responses to such situations. In the future, I think the most important thing to do when a similar situation arises, is to analyse it in the same manner. This will allow me to reconsider and consolidate my views on how I respond to the death of patients, making future events easier to deal with.

COMMENTS ON REFLECTION

This is a good piece of reflection. The author sets the scene, sensitively describes the sort of patient he is clerking and her social circumstances, and confides in the reader that at one stage he wished he could go home rather than try to get a history from this hearing-impaired woman. He established a good rapport and relationship with the patient, making her death a very painful and poignant experience for him.

He explains his emotions of shock, guilt and helplessness when he discovers her death and has good insight into his inexperience with coping with the death of patients he has clerked. He quite justifiably feels professionally satisfied that he performed well and the experience will be helpful for his education and career.

COMMENTS ON ENGLISH

What was done well

➤ The general quality of the English here is very good. The vocabulary is carefully chosen to increase the clarity of the situation and emotions described, which makes for a pleasant and interesting reading experience. Some areas of the essay are also effectively punctuated and this adds pace and meaning to the reflection. The third paragraph is particularly strong; the following is an exemplary extract that demonstrates an excellent use of the colon (to introduce a list) and the semicolon (to separate more wordy items on a list):

I also felt a sense of guilt for several reasons: guilt at the fact that I had not seen her closer to the time of her death; guilt that I had not found out about her death earlier/checked her progress more recently; guilt that perhaps I had not picked up on some symptoms or signs that may have alerted medics to her imminent deterioration; guilt that I was not more upset.

The way the student uses punctuation to break down a series of complex emotions is incredibly effective as it allows the reader to track their feelings and thus engage emotionally with the reflection. The repetition of the word "guilt" is also striking and emphasises the student's overriding concerns.

What could have been done better

➤ Whilst most of the English here is good, the student often misuses commas. You rarely need to use commas before or after the words "and" or "because" as these words are connectives; you should never use these words to start a sentence either. The student frequently and unnecessarily uses commas after the word "and".

Over the past few months I have reflected on many important issues and questions that I have been faced with, however one recent event has stood out. Whilst on take at the Whittington Hospital, I was asked by the Registrar to clerk a young lady (21 year old) in the acute admissions unit (AAU) who had had a small amount of vomiting and haemetemesis. I approached the patient and asked for permission to speak to her about why she came to Hospital. Although she gave permission, I did get the sense that she was a bit anxious. The consultation started in the typical way and I built a good rapport with the patient. About 10 minutes into the consultation whilst finishing the 'History of Presenting Complaint' section, the patient unexpectedly started to cry. I asked whether everything was ok and whether there was something particular that was upsetting her. She didn't reply. I suggested she lay down on the bed and offered to get a doctor or nurse. She said no, got her emotions together again and said she was ready to carry on. I asked whether she wanted some time alone and that I could come back a bit later, however she insisted that I carry on with my questions. Apprehensively I continued with my questions but pointed out that if at any time she wanted to stop, she just had to ask. The rest of the consultation continued as normal, however when I asked to examine her at the end, she looked nervous and anxious again and although she did give permission I did not feel it was appropriate and so thanked her and said that once I had spoken to the team someone would come to see her. I reported back to the Registrar who said that her GP had phoned and said there was quite a big anxiety issue. I later accompanied the Registrar who saw the patient, and after a quick consultation said she could go home and needed no further investigation/treatment. The patient was extremely happy to hear this news and thanked the Registrar and me as we left the room.

Later that day I spent some time reflecting on my experience. My initial reaction when the patient started to cry was shock. I had never seen a patient have a breakdown in front of me, and definitely wasn't expecting it from the brief history that I had been given by the Registrar. I feel that once the breakdown had happened I reacted appropriately and offered to get someone, to leave her alone for a little while or stay with her. She wanted me to stay. The rapport, which I had previously built, definitely helped the patient during the breakdown and after a minute she was calm again. Although this patient wanted me to stay, I can appreciate that a different patient may have wanted to be alone for a few moments or may have wanted to see a doctor, and that their wishes should be respected.

I have asked myself whether, having suspected when I first met the patient that she seemed anxious, I should have come back later, rather than start the consultation. Having thought a great deal about this I feel that it was the correct choice to start the consultation, as the patient may have just wanted to speak to someone. Additionally, most patients are anxious by being in Hospital and eventually finding out their diagnosis will likely give them the ability to process and deal with the anxiety.

I chose not to examine her as I got the sense that she may have another breakdown and so thought it was better to wait for a doctor to examine her. Looking back I still feel this was the appropriate choice of action, however I have wondered how I would deal with this situation if I were a FY1, and would have to examine her. She did give consent and was not coerced into this, so that is not an issue, however she clearly felt apprehensive. Although I would be concerned that she may have another breakdown, I believe that I would perform the examination but take extra care to be sensitive to her feelings, and explain exactly what I was doing to, as much as possible, put her mind at ease.

Another issue arising from this situation is should the Registrar have warned me that there was an anxiety issue, or should I have been the first one to speak to her. I think that the Registrar most likely forgot about the anxiety issue when he asked me to speak to her. Alternatively, perhaps he wanted me to experience a difficult consultation. The latter does raise a duty of care issue. The General Medical Council say that the care of the patient should be the first concern, and not my education. Although I did get permission to speak to the patient, should I have been put in that situation, or rather should it have been a more experienced member of the team who spoke to her?

This experience has shown me an additional benefit of building a good rapport with the patient. I have also learnt that as a doctor I will have to expect the unexpected and be ready to deal with constantly changing situations and environments. If in the future I am faced with a similar situation, I feel that I would be better prepared and have less initial shock. I would quickly assess the situation, evaluating what would be in the patient's best interest and take appropriate action, thereby offering a better standard of care.

COMMENTS ON REFLECTION

This has all the ingredients of a good reflective essay. The scene is set clearly and simply; the author captures the picture of an anxious, tearful young woman and has good insight into his actions, what he did and what he chose not to do. He also puts himself in the position of a Foundation Year 1 Doctor (FY1) doctor who has to complete the clerking to get a diagnosis and plan management. He includes reflection-in-action and detailed reflection-on-action. His conclusions are sound and sensible.

COMMENTS ON ENGLISH
What was done well

➤ This essay is mostly very well written. It is well structured and punctuated and therefore easy to follow and engage with. Important sentences are short and powerful and break up the writing effectively. Good writing will often contain a pertinent mixture of short and long sentences. The short sentences act as powerful breaks to the writing and can therefore be used to convey interesting or important information. A particularly good extract that demonstrates effective variation of sentence length and structure is: "About 10 minutes into the consultation whilst finishing the 'History of Presenting Complaint' section, the patient unexpectedly started to cry. I asked whether everything was ok and whether there was something particular that was upsetting her. She didn't reply."

What could have been done better

> Whilst most of the writing is of a high quality, certain sentences are awkwardly phrased. Medical students often overcomplicate sentences that contain important revelations or complex issues. Remember, just because the content is complex, the phrasing should not have to be. The following is an example of this:

Original student version

Another issue arising from this situation is should the Registrar have warned me that there was an anxiety issue, or should I have been the first one to speak to her.

Amended version

I am not sure if the registrar should have warned me about her anxiety or even if I, as a student, should have been the first to speak with her.

I have decided to write upon my experience during the Surgery module where I was on 'night-take' from 8pm to 8am with a fellow student. I was attached to the surgical FY2 doctor on call that night and have chosen to reflect upon this experience as it is on this occasion where I felt I learned some of the most important lessons so far in medicine. The two specific experiences that will be discussed include: the manner in which dealing with a worried patient and their distressed family as well as the understanding that doctors should increasingly involve patients in their own management and care. Both of these reflections are centred upon one particular patient that arrived at A&E earlier that day.

The first patient we saw that night was SP, a 21 year old black female who had presented with severe abdominal pain and fever in the afternoon, with results later confirming renal colic and septicaemia. However, her medical history was complex as she suffered from sarcoidosis from a young age and had since experienced numerous complications such as hepatomegaly and splenomegaly as well as blindness in her left eye. Her situation had since improved from the afternoon and she was in a stable condition when we saw her. The family were present with her and were understandably very anxious about the situation.

Firstly, I am going to discuss the experience of dealing with a worried patient and their distressed family members. The FY2 doctor was, in my opinion, thoroughly impressive in the way he dealt with the situation in a calm and professional yet highly reassuring and supportive manner. As I watched him carry out his history and examination, I recall him gaining all the necessary information as any standard FY2 doctor would. It was only when the patient became very worried when he told her she had kidney stones (resulting in septicaemia) that I realised the great professional manner he had about him.

When I recall this incident, I realise the importance of gaining the trust and confidence of the patient and their family. When SP asked the FY2 questions about what renal colic was, he was able to explain it well in very simple terms and took time to sit with the patient and make sure she was completely aware of what her body was doing in response to it. I am sure that if I had been asked that same question, I would not have been able to describe it as well as he did without using medical jargon which could have unnecessarily confused and frightened the family. Furthermore, when the family became increasingly distressed and started to demand that the doctor and hospital take the very best care of their daughter, I distinctly remember feeling very nervous and not knowing what to say if I was in the FY2's situation. However, he again responded in a reassuring manner without giving false hope and took time to answer their concerns rather than rushing off to see the next patient. After observing this incident, I have learned the importance of being able to explain complicated scenarios in a simple and caring manner with the aim of gaining the trust and confidence of the patient and their family.

The second recollection I will discuss is the realisation that patients should be increasingly involved in their own management as they often know their condition and bodies much better than the medical staff attending to them. In this particular case, as SP had lived with sarcoidosis from early childhood and had experienced numerous complications, she knew a lot about the disease itself and the way her body dealt with it from her regular hospital visits. For example, SP told the doctor what her normal observations were (e.g. HR, BP) so this made his job much easier in determining what was abnormal and what areas needed special attention. When I accompanied the doctor to take a blood culture sample from her later in the night, she told us that she only has one successful vein for taking blood in her frequent experience of attending hospitals. However, he dismissed her advice and attempted other veins first, which I agreed with as there appeared to be more suitable alternatives. Ironically, after 3 unsuccessful attempts at two different sites, he resorted to trying the vein she suggested and was able to get an immediate blood sample.

This incident, although minor in nature, taught me that medical staff should not underestimate the knowledge of the patient as they often know best about their bodies. I am glad to have observed this as next time I will be sure to listen to the patient thoroughly and take their advice into strong consideration before opting to act in my own accordance. Reflecting upon this event has allowed me to understand the importance of an inclusive attitude towards patients rather than a paternalistic 'I know better' attitude, the latter of which is still in use by some within the medical community. I am now much more supportive of the view held by the GMC whereby they encourage doctors to 'work in partnership' with their patients.

Overall, my experience on night take was very useful and informative. It was the first time I really felt I was undertaking actual medicine as part of a 'team', for example by clerking patients and taking numerous blood samples. Having reflected on such incidents as discussed above, I feel more confident and aware of the skills and attributes necessary to improve myself as a doctor and make the experience for the patient and their family one of trust and reassurance. These will undoubtedly stand me in good stead and will hopefully allow me to develop into a better doctor and improve the care of my future patients.

COMMENTS ON REFLECTION

This reflective piece is poor in a number of ways. There is excessive description; the first two paragraphs could be deleted without any loss of understanding of the event. How much description should there be in a reflective essay? Enough to allow the reader to understand the scenario the author is reflecting on and why it was a significant experience for the author. The introduction and description of the scene and people involved should be written concisely and with sufficient detail to transport the reader to the setting.

The author also tries to deal with two issues rather than sticking to one and, unfortunately, does neither justice. He writes that the Foundation Year 2 (FY2) doctor had a great "professional manner about him" but does not explore what he thought was "great" about this manner, losing an opportunity for reflecting on an important and interesting subject for reflection: role-modelling. Medicine is in many respects an apprenticeship and, as in other professions and types of work, our behaviour, attitudes and practice are based on the characteristics of our teachers and peers who lead and teach us. We all learn something from the people we work with: their dress sense, their voice, presentation, approach, communication style and manners with patients and colleagues; their sense of humour or lack of it; their sense of decency, fair play, generosity; their teaching skills, technical or operating skills, attitude to work, colleagues, work–life balance, study skills, analytical skills and political views. Which of these or other characteristics did the author think the FY2 had and why? Which ones did the FY2 not have? How did the FY2 inspire the author or give him a new perspective about medicine and how he might practise it? Does the author believe or consider that he learned something important from the FY2?

The penultimate and final paragraphs are when most reflective essays provide the reader with reflection, although as we have pointed out in other essays reflection need not be restricted to the end, and can and should be introduced throughout the essay. When we arrive at the end of this essay we are disappointed. We are given superficial reflection: "next time I will", and a perfunctory, unnecessary and unhelpful reference to the General Medical Council guidelines. The author has not reflected to any depth about his night "on take" and the reader is left thinking whether at this stage the author has thought about this experience, has learned anything at all from it or, indeed, has the capacity to learn from his clinical experiences.

This unsatisfactory standard of reflection is unfortunately all too common in junior students. It is a good example of how not to write a reflective piece and that is why we have included it. Reflection is about observation, thought, insight, analysis and sensible, honest conclusions that will take you forward personally and professionally.

COMMENTS ON ENGLISH
What was done well
➤ The general quality of the writing here is not bad at all. The sentences and paragraphs are logically ordered and structured and most parts of the essay make sense. Most of the sentences here are simply constructed and may seem basic, yet this style is preferable to long, rambling sentences that often sound either unrefined and sloppy or pretentious and verbose. If in doubt, keep it simple.

What could have been done better
➤ Whilst the essay is easy to follow, parts are too schematic and clumsy. Sentences such as "Firstly, I am going to discuss the experience of dealing with a worried patient and their distressed family members" and "The second recollection I will discuss is the realisation that patients should be increasingly involved in their own management" are unnecessary. Do not say what you are going to say: just say it!

Spanish is spoken by a large fraction of New York's inhabitants. Indeed, it is often their only language. Particularly elderly persons often only have a very limited command of the English language. The segregation between English and Spanish speakers is pretty impressive. In the lab in which I worked, all the academic staff and students spoke immaculate English. But to communicate with the support staff, the cleaners, the plumbers, and even the lab assistants, I had to switch to Spanish, English really wasn't an option. In fact, much of New York's lower social class is Hispanic and speaks Spanish.

The large majority of people presenting in the emergency room is of course Spanish, as their inability to pay for insurance forces them to use the ER as a make-shift GP practice. Yet, the majority of doctors in the ER are white and middle-class. They speak English, not Spanish, and their command of Spanish is often miserable at best.

Thus, communication between patients and doctors is on average pretty awful. Sign language only goes so far. How do you ask about the character of pain with your hands? This problem has of course been recognised. Health professionals are encouraged to learn Spanish, speaking Spanish is certainly a plus in the recruitment, and there is a translator available at all times.

Nevertheless, I very frequently found myself helping to mediate between a doctor and a patient. In fact, I was often sent out to clerk a patient and then present them to the doctors, precisely because I spoke Spanish. I would then present the patient to the English-speaking doctor, and then return with further questions. For me, this process was of course great, as it allowed me to clerk patients in detail, to be part of the medical process, and to practise my Spanish. But patients know quite well what role I was playing, and they really wanted to speak to the doctor, not to me, the student, or indeed to the translator.

The main doctor I shadowed was Dr. XX, who is Hispanic himself. A number of times, I would have clerked a patient for one of the younger doctors on his team. If there were any questions, he would of course come and review the patient himself.

It was just so often striking to see how much more patients were willing to tell him, how much clinically highly relevant information they just volunteered when faced with a person of their own ethnic group with whom there were neither cultural nor language communication barriers.

There are too many of these experiences to enumerate them. They have clearly shown to me that it is crucial that the health work force should be ethnically matched to the patient population; and that doctors should make a particular effort to minimize cultural barriers. One relatively straightforward way to do so is to learn the language their patients speak.

COMMENTS ON REFLECTION

This is not a reflective piece. The author describes rather vaguely, from his Emergency Room experience in New York City, the communication problems that may exist if Spanish patients cannot understand a doctor who does not speak Spanish. He gives no evidence for his assertion. The author does not provide a specific clinical example illustrating his belief; he states that there were too many examples to "enumerate" (this is in fact a misuse of the word and he probably means cite). For the purposes of a reflective essay this is *precisely* what he should have done. We see nothing of the author beyond description of his place in these events and we see nothing of a real patient–doctor interaction. The author might have been able to cite an example of Dr XXXX extracting a key point from the clinical history that fundamentally changed the management of a Spanish-speaking patient who could not explain something to a non-Spanish-speaking doctor. This could have been followed by an exploration of the event and the author could have related how he felt, what it meant to him and what he learned from it. The author also advocates that doctors should learn the language of the patient they see. This would not be practical for doctors working in a European town or city where there are people from many different countries speaking different languages. For example, in Tower Hamlets, East London, the local community hospital provides care for people speaking over 50 different languages.

COMMENTS ON ENGLISH

What was done well

➤ Parts of this essay contain very effectively structured and varied sentences that maintain pace and the reader's interest. A particularly good trio of sentences reads: "Thus, communication between patients and doctors is on average pretty awful. Sign language only goes so far. How do you ask about the character of pain with your hands?" Here the student has started with a slightly longer sentence, followed by a short, factual statement, which is then followed by a rhetorical question. Incorporating these simple, grammatical features makes your writing more interesting to read.

What could have been done better

➤ Tense confusion: The student dabbles between tenses in the opening paragraph, which is rather disorienting and unsettling for the reader. It is important to write your essay in a consistent way; using the past tense to recount experiences is preferable. Whilst you might want to reflect in the present tense and ponder future practice in the future tense, past experiences are often best written in the past tense. The key thing to remember is to keep the tenses consistent.

Original student version

I had to switch to Spanish, English really wasn't an option. In fact, much of New York's lower social class is Hispanic and speaks Spanish.

Amended version
Speaking English would not have been helpful because most of New York's lower social classes speak Spanish.

➤ Clichés and truisms: When reflecting on a particularly poignant and important issue, you should endeavour to make your writing as original and succinct as possible. Phrases such as "English really wasn't an option" and "their command of Spanish is often miserable at best" are clichéd and imprecise. Better and more informative replacements could be: "Speaking English was a potentially unproductive solution", "speaking English would not have been helpful or beneficial" and "their spoken Spanish was inadequate". These phrases are more specific and therefore explain the situation more clearly.

My first attempt at cannulation came late on in my surgical rotation at the Royal Free. It wasn't that I had actively avoided performing cannulation over the previous eight weeks, but the thought certainly made me nervous. I had heard stories from other students about their own trials and tribulations with the cannula needle and however much I practised on the plastic model arms in the clinical skills centre, I never really felt fully-prepared to try and have a go on a real, living patient.

Finally, during my Critical Care Placement, I was given the opportunity to cannulate a patient in A&E. The clinical skills tutor had brought two other students and myself to the department and had left us to decide who would cannulate the first patient. Neither of my colleagues jumped at the chance, so I nervously put myself forward, fully aware that there would be few better opportunities to practise on a patient.

With my equipment set up, we went to meet the patient who, we were told, was brought to the hospital following an episode of haemoptysis. We would have to wear face masks to see him. We stepped into the room to meet the patient, who swayed drowsily in his seat as he struggled to stay upright, and his brother who accompanied him. I quickly introduced myself and explained what I was going to do. I felt as though I were in autopilot mode: my well-rehearsed words came out smoothly even though my heart was racing. My equipment was already prepared and there was no delaying the inevitable any longer. It wasn't until I knelt down to try and find a vein that I realised exactly how different it was compared to practising on the models: the patient was not only slightly overweight, but a thick covering of hair obscured most visible traces of the vessels in his arm. Even with the tourniquet in place, I couldn't find anything. The clinical skills tutor saw me struggling and took over, promptly locating a suitable vein for me to try. I squared up the needle and was mortified to see my fingers shaking considerably. I took some deep breaths, and desperately tried to steady myself before pushing it into the arm. There was no flashback, just a small wince of pain from the patient, who was looking increasingly drowsy. As I withdrew the cannula, the patient began to look very faint, and had to be helped to the floor.

I felt very self-conscious. I felt as though I had made the patient suffer unduly in my nervous attempt to cannulate him. He was helped up onto the bed, and the clinical skills tutor asked me whether I wanted to have another try. Although I would have liked at that moment to escape, I went against my immediate inclincation and accepted the offer, quickly preparing my equipment once more. The second attempt wasn't quite as shaky as the first, and thankfully it was successful. I remember the sense of relief and pride that I felt when I saw the flashback of blood.

When I look back at these events, I realise a few things: firstly, although practising clinical skills outside of the clinical setting is useful for learning a technique, it is no substitution for learning in the context of the real patient. There are so many more variables in the hospital that cannot necessarily be rehearsed or even anticipated. In a clinical context, there is automatically a lot more pressure on you to perform well, especially when you are being observed not only by the patient, but also by their relatives and your own colleagues and superiors. Communicating with the patient, to explain procedures to them and to comfort them, is also integral to the whole experience. And all the while you may have to contend with your own nerves, the unfamiliar setting and the patient's worsening condition.

Given all of these factors, it seems to me that I – and indeed anyone wishing to work in the medical profession – must endeavour to put myself out, to bite the bullet, and seize the opportunities to practise these clinical skills when they present themselves. I think there is a tendency amongst many medical students – one with which I can easily identify - to sit back and allow others to step forward. I recognise the fact that I tend to shy away from situations when I am put on the spot, in which I might be made to look foolish. Part of the problem is that I carry high expectations for myself: like everyone else, I have had to prove myself academically to get to where I am. The trouble is that so much of medicine is practical in nature: it cannot be learned purely through book work. In order to acquire the necessary skills I must be prepared to have a go, to risk embarrassing myself or messing up, so that I can learn from my mistakes and improve.

At the end of the day, I am still a student! I am here to learn: I am not expected to know everything, nor am I expected to be an expert in performing clinical skills on my first attempt. However, I will not always be a doctor-in-training: one day I *will* be expected, and relied upon, to perform these skills accurately and confidently. It therefore strikes me that the supportive environment of the teaching hospital is the perfect one in which to practise and learn. I therefore hope that in future I might take a more proactive view towards learning the practical skills that will be required of me, in the same way that I already try to approach my academic studies. I hope that I will be prepared to accept the possibility that I might not get it right first time, but that at least by trying I will learn something, and that it will become easier and easier with each attempt.

COMMENTS ON REFLECTION

This is a well-written essay (apart from one or two clichés) and is a very good example of high-quality reflection. The author's anxiety and insecurity is well described in the first half. The second half of the essay shows good insight. The reader is left in no doubt that the author has gone through quite an emotional and educational experience with this clinical encounter and will be a better technical practitioner and doctor because of it and his reflection. He touches on communication with patients, the importance of gaining real clinical experience and his own reluctance to do things to spare his embarrassment when he makes mistakes. This is the fundamental importance of reflective practice.

COMMENTS ON ENGLISH
What was done well

➤ This essay is structured in a coherent and logical way, making it easy for the reader to follow. The fluent writing style, which draws upon a good range of appropriate vocabulary, also enhances the reading experience. On the whole, despite a few grammatical problems, this essay is well written and enjoyable to read.

What could have been done better

➤ Whilst this essay is very well written, it demonstrates a few grammatical errors. One such error involves erroneous pronouns. Many students confuse the "me", "myself" and "I" pronouns. If in doubt over which pronoun to use, try removing the other person from the sentence and see what fits best; reordering the sentence could be necessary. In the following example, "myself" is used instead of "me". If we remove "two other students and" from the sentence it would read: "The clinical skills tutor had brought myself to the department and had left us to decide who would cannulate the first patient", which obviously sounds incorrect.

Original student version

The clinical skills tutor had brought two other students and myself to the department and had left us to decide who would cannulate the first patient.

Amended version

The clinical skills tutor had brought me and two other students to the department and had left us to decide who would cannulate the first patient.

➤ Although this student is clearly an able writer, they do include a few clichés that detract from the quality of their work. Phrases such as "trials and tribulations", "bite the bullet" and "jumped at the chance" are bland and could be more effectively articulated with more original language.
➤ This essay is generally well punctuated but the student uses many dashes, which are too informal for a piece of academic work. The dashes could easily be replaced with sets of bracketing commas, which effectively function like brackets but in a less divisive way:

Original student version

Given all of these factors, it seems to me that I – and indeed anyone wishing to work in the medical profession – must endeavour to put myself out, to bite the bullet, and seize the opportunities to practise these clinical skills when they present themselves. I think there is a tendency amongst many medical students – one with which I can easily identify – to sit back and allow others to step forward.

Amended version

Given all of these factors, it seems to me that I, and indeed anyone wishing to work in the medical profession, must endeavour to put myself out, to bite the bullet, and seize the opportunities to practise these clinical skills when they present themselves. I think there is a tendency amongst many medical students, one with which I can easily identify, to sit back and allow others to step forward.

It is expected that possible management decisions regarding a patient's healthcare will be discussed, debated or can even be disagreed upon by healthcare professionals before being presented to the patient. As a medical student, it is commonplace to not understand the decisions made over a management plan, especially when the patient has a condition that you have not experienced or read about. However, there are situations when, despite the relative inexperience of medical students, we feel that the plan is not appropriate and this leaves us wondering what to do. I would like to reflect on such a situation that I have experienced.

Having taken a full history and examined a 21 year old woman, I was confused by her clinical picture and sought help from a junior doctor on the ward. She had presented with mild right iliac fossa pain, renal colic and haematuria and we discussed various differential diagnoses involving various renal, urinary, gynaecological and gastro-intestinal causes. On the following ward round my consultant (surgeon) explained that appendicitis seemed likely and that she should have surgery. I was surprised to hear this, especially given that the patient had had very few investigations done, and upon asking the surgeon about this decision he explained that he had seen countless appendicitis's in his experience and that, although atypical, this was very likely to be appendicitis. It later became apparent that the patient had not been seen by a gynaecologist and had only had a KUB X-ray to rule out ureteric stones, but no other imaging. The following day I found out that the patient had turned out to have an ovarian cyst and having followed her up later, found her very disappointed to have a new and unnecessary scar on her abdomen.

After my initial surprise at hearing the management plan, the consultants' justification of his decision put my mind at rest over the matter; I had after all had very little experience of the condition and I was in no position at that time to put up any opposition. However, after the following day I was left unsure of what think; had the consultant made the wrong decision or the right one, but been unlucky? Ultimately, I questioned whether I should have said something at the time and whether the eventual outcome was avoidable. Having said this, the outcome for the patient was not that bad and her care was swiftly passed to the gynaecologists. The ultimate outcome for me was confusion, the situation raising issues in my mind about my role as a medical student, but also my relationship to consultants.

As a medical student, my involvement with the patient's care was a learning exercise in both my skills in patient interaction when I initially clerked her, but also in learning about appendicitis through the consultants actions. As I alluded to early, being relatively inexperienced, I generally assume the consultant is correct all the time and resign my understanding to his/her decisions. However, whilst I feel that it was good that I raised my initial concerns; I did not ultimately raise enough concerns or be convincing enough to stimulate the surgeon to do further investigations. Whether I should have pushed my point further to get my point across is certainly worth exploring.

It is important to highlight that medical students do not have (or perhaps should not need to have) a duty of care to patients when it comes to their management plans, and for that reason I had no duty to push my point further with my consultant. However, in the interest of trying to be a good student and trying to learn exactly what is happening with the patient and why such decisions are being made, it is important to always be inquisitive and ask relevant questions. This may well have led to the consultant reconsidering his/her decision. For this reason, I feel now that I should have questioned further. As well as this, in the interest of being a good person, it is important to raise any issues that one feels might significantly affect the patient.

So, why did I not say more at the time? And what factors were inhibiting me? In short it comes down to a lack of confidence in my own knowledge (perhaps rightly so) and the fact that as a student I have to be able to get along with my consultant to be able to get the most out of a 9 week rotation. As well as this, my consultant grades my activities within his/her firm, a grade which contributes to my end of year mark. For that reason it is important to make good impression and not to waste the consultant's time on a busy ward-round, especially having already asked several questions.

To conclude it is important to weigh up whether I did indeed act appropriately or whether I should have done more. It is also worth considering whether I now feel that the consultant made the correct decision. Looking back, I feel that my decision to act should have come down to a judgment about the consultant's character and the importance of the issue. For that reason, I feel that I should have raised my further concerns, but perhaps after the ward round, or even via a trusted registrar to avoid unnecessary backlash or indeed embarrassment for myself. The issue of whether the consultant made the right choice to operate is much harder to resolve. The fact of the matter is that my consultant may have previously seen very similar appendicitis presentations to this patient, but that a gynaecological surgeon may have previously seen very similar presentations of an ovarian cyst to this patient and the diagnosis could have gone either way. Whilst one could argue that it would not have done harm to do further investigations, an important take home message from this experience is that medicine is by no means a clear cut science and a diagnosis is never set in stone.

COMMENTS ON REFLECTION

The author has described the clinical scenario briefly and reflected on his inexperience and his wish not to irritate the consultant by questioning his clinical diagnosis of appendicitis. During training as a medical student and beyond, there will be many similar situations where a more senior doctor makes a decision with which the student or trainee may disagree. This is a good focus for a formal reflection as it is a complex situation; there is no simple method for sorting out such dilemmas. It would be interesting to read the consultant's reflection of this incident and whether the student's question seeded any doubts in his mind about appendicectomy.

The author has reflected well and honestly, stating his inexperience and his embarrassment about questioning the consultant too much, and compromising his firm's end-of-year mark. His final paragraph has insight and maturity.

COMMENTS ON ENGLISH

What was done well

➤ This essay is well structured and fluently written. Part of this is due to how well it has been paragraphed; each paragraph reflects a shift in time or subject and they are excellently linked, thematically and grammatically. A particular strength of the paragraphs is how each opens. The opening line of each paragraph strongly and effectively sets the tone of what is to follow. This type of paragraph opening is sometimes called a "topic sentence". Topic sentences subtly outline the purpose of the paragraph and keep your writing focused. If you are prone to sprawling, unfocused paragraphs, then starting each one with a topic sentence could be a good idea. Examples of good topic sentences in this essay include: "As a medical student, my involvement with the patient's care was a learning exercise", "So, why did I not say more at the time?" and "To conclude . . .". Note how each of these sentences/sentence openings influence the content of the paragraph they begin.

What could have been done better

➤ Whilst most of this essay is well punctuated, there is a misplaced apostrophe and this has very confusing consequences. The student has placed the apostrophe after the "s" instead of before the "s" of "consultants", which makes the doctor plural, allowing the reader to think the decision referred to was a group decision, not the decision of one individual:

Original student version

After my initial surprise at hearing the management plan, the consultants' justification of his decision put my mind at rest over the matter.

Amended version

After my initial surprise at hearing the management plan, the consultant's justification of his decision put my mind at rest.

A lot of doctors claim to be effective communicators. Or are they? It seems that relaying and passing on information to patients has become more challenging nowadays. This is partly due to the fact that London has become one of the most multicultural and multidisciplinary capitals of the world. And also, due to the fact that medicine has moved from a "paternalistic" status to a more "self taking decisions about care" status, with increasing need for more interpersonal communication. Hence, one could argue that communication skills, within medicine, have evolved through the years and have become one of the most important aspects of care that patients are offered within the NHS in the UK. And how does that translate for doctors and even more for medical students? Practise, practise, practise!

It is hard to take complete medical history from competent patients that are able to talk and give information for themselves. It is even more challenging to take medical history from people who can't talk or are not competent. It happened that I had such a challenging acquaintance when I clerked Mrs S. During my study of the COOP module, I had to present a patient as a key student during bedside teaching. So I went to the hospital to find a patient to talk to and take their medical history. I wasn't sure which patient was appropriate to clerk, so I asked one of the Specialist Registrars (SpR) to recommend a patient with a good clinical history. The SpR recommended that I clerked Mrs S. At the time, I had no idea who Mrs S. was or what her health status was like. But I assumed that since the SpR recommended her, she would have been a competent patient from which I could have taken a straight-forward history. As soon as I reached Mrs S.'s room, I checked that I was at the correct room and I looked inside to make a first assessment of my patient. As I looked inside the room, I couldn't believe my eyes. I checked again the room number and still couldn't believe my eyes. In the room, I could see an elderly lady that was extremely debilitated because of severe Rheumatoid Arthritis (RA), with unbelievable muscle wasting -for the fact that she was a patient in a British hospital in the 21st century- with severe hand deformities and a tracheostomy applied to her neck with a speech valve. I immediately thought that it would be very difficult for me to take medical history from Mrs S. because she would have been exhausted by the time I finished talking to her, as it must have been very difficult for her to talk with the speech valve. Also, I assumed that she wasn't fully competent by the look of her physical appearance. I felt kind of "betrayed". Why was the SpR so mean to me in order to send me to clerk a non-competent patient that is not able to talk properly and would have taken me hours to take a proper history from Mrs S.? I felt rather stupid for not reading Mrs S.'s notes before hand and for blindly following the SpR's indications for the "perfect" clinical history.

But then I thought even if it was difficult to clerk Mrs S., I wanted to give it a try. I approached Mrs S. and introduced myself as a medical student. At the time, she was listening to the radio and as soon as she saw me in the room, she shut the radio down and put it on the table beside her. She nodded her head to salute me. Then I explained to her that I wanted to talk to her about her health and what has brought her to the hospital. She immediately nodded her head, showing that she understood everything I told her and I immediately started to realise that I was wrong to assume just by her appearance that she was not competent. As I explained to Mrs S. that everything she told me was confidential, I took her permission and started asking her questions.

She started talking, but no voice was coming out of her mouth, since she had bilateral vocal cord palsy, And the situation was even more complicated as she couldn't use her speech valve because it was very painful to use, since she had laryngitis. And even if she used the speech valve, her sayings couldn't reach my ears because the infection in her throat debilitated her speech and gave her a hoarse voice. At the beginning she was talking slowly and I was just able to read her lips. But as the conversation went on she was too fast for me to keep up. So, I gave her my notepad and asked her if she could write what she tried to tell me. The conversation really went on smoothly. I was really impressed by her excellent hearing and mental capacity. I got al the medical details from Mrs S. and we even had a "social" talk about her life and she even asked me questions about my course and my hometown.At the end of the conversation I thanked her, and took her permission to present her case to my colleagues during bedside teaching.

After I left her room I thought of how well the conversation went with Mrs S. and how polite she was to me, even though she was really ill. Also, I realised how wrong I was by judging Mrs S.'s competence just by her physical appearance and to doubt my SpR's choice for sending me to take Mrs S.'s medical history. I was really satisfied and proud of myself that I talked to Mrs S and didn't run away as soon as I've seen her. Finally, I've learnt a valuable lesson; that physical incapacity is not always accompanied by mental incapacity, and Mrs S was a true story of that.

COMMENTS ON REFLECTION

Nearly all of this essay is descriptive and this is disappointing. There is an insignificant piece of reflection in the final paragraph when the author congratulates himself on his efforts rather than purposefully reflecting on the experience. His concluding sentence is something that most people would understand without having any medical education. The author's claimed enthusiasm for good communication skills in medicine is not supported by this piece of writing: he does not describe the content of the "conversation" he had with the patient, only the difficulties in conducting it. He does describe having a "social" talk: what does he mean by this? In this piece he could have shared his feelings at meeting the patient, how he felt about older people being unable to communicate in a straightforward way, the difficulties of having a tracheostomy and what problems the patient had, and how these impacted on him. What did he learn from this case other than making assumptions based on appearance? How can this experience help him deal with other patients who cannot communicate clearly? What will he do the next time he has a similar patient? There was a lot more he could have reflected on and communicated to the reader. He briefly suggests some understanding of the registrar's aim in advising him to see this patient. Again this could have been usefully explored further.

COMMENTS ON ENGLISH
What was done well

➤ This essay is well structured in terms of its paragraphs and its sentences. The latter vary in length and format effectively to add meaning and pace. When you write extended pieces of work like reflective essays, it is important that your writing maintains momentum. Sentences that are all too long, all too short or monotonously constructed can detract from descriptions of even the most exciting or tense moments in surgery. Whether you use rhetorical questions, repeat certain words or simply contrast longer, descriptive sentences alongside shorter, revelatory ones, some kind of variety is key. Extracts that are particularly strong for this reason include:

Hence, one could argue that communication skills, within medicine, have evolved through the years and have become one of the most important aspects of care that patients are offered within the NHS in the UK. And how does that translate for doctors and even more for medical students? Practise, practise, practise!

She nodded her head to salute me. Then I explained to her that I wanted to talk to her about her health and what has brought her to the hospital. She immediately nodded her head, showing that she understood everything I told her and I immediately started to realise that I was wrong to assume just by her appearance that she was not competent.

What could have been done better

➤ Most English-language academics will tell you to never start a sentence with the word "and". The word "and" is a connective word and should only be used to link two clauses together within a sentence. Whilst media texts may feature sentences that begin with "and", it is almost never advisable to begin sentences in more formal writing this way. Starting with "and" also makes the sentence sound like an afterthought, detracting from its importance. The following two sentences, which both appear in the first paragraph and feature an unnecessary and erroneous "and", could have been changed easily:

Original student version
This is partly due to the fact that London has become one of the most multicultural and multidisciplinary capitals of the world. And also, due to the fact that medicine has moved from a "paternalistic" status . . .

Amended version
This is partly due to the fact that London has become one of the most multicultural and multidisciplinary capitals of the world. It is also due to the fact that medicine has moved from a "paternalistic" status . . .

Original student version
Hence, one could argue that communication skills, within medicine, have evolved through the years and have become one of the most important aspects of care that patients are offered within the NHS in the UK. And how does that translate for doctors and even more for medical students?

Amended version

Hence, one could argue that in medicine, communication skills have evolved and have become one of the most important aspects of care that patients are offered within the NHS. How does that translate for doctors and medical students?

A particular incident has remained with me over the course of the past couple of weeks. My firm had just begun the Surgery module which I had been looking forward to as it is of particular interest to me. However, I had been particularly concerned about starting this module. So far into my medical studentship, theatres had been quite a hostile environment. As a student I'd always felt in the way- or that I shouldn't be there and that I was a hindrance to staff and the convalescence of the patient.

I had, therefore, reservations about entering theatres on only the second day of the new module. Pushing my way through the heavy theatre doors with 5 other medical students, I anticipated the familiar avoidance of the theatre staff, the gruff acknowledgement of the surgeon and then to be told to stay in a far corner to be avoided for the next couple of hours. On entering the theatres, the scenario couldn't have been more different. To my surprise the main operating surgeon welcomed us all in and without hesitation asked a senior registrar to explain to us the surgery he was finishing. Relief washed through me. The team explained that they had been expecting us and were immediately engaged in learning about the procedure. We watched as the operation was finished. Just before the patient was closed the surgeon turned to us, and with a smile, asked enthusiastically: "which of you would like to learn to suture?"

I immediately jumped at the opportunity to suture. Due to previous theatre experience I had never been offered such an opportunity before and had to explain numerous times that I was a novice, as I was sure I had misunderstood such a generous offer. The surgeon took it with good humour and explained that I would be guided through it thoroughly and that the patient had fully consented to students being present and that this was within the remit of the consent procedure.

An issue of much concern had switched to become the best day of learning for me to date. The opportunity I was given by the surgeon, his team and the patient to learn such a valuable practical skill was remarkable, and one which I didn't take for granted. Every student was engaged in some activity that day, but most importantly was encouraged to be involved at some level.

This event has allowed me to reflect upon a number of issues within the medical profession, including teamwork, education and respect for patient autonomy.

A major point of reflection for me was that of the master/apprentice relationship between the students and the surgeons that day. The fact that they were prepared to put time aside to teach us which in turn enabled us to open up and absorb information in an unthreatening environment. This encouraged us to participate, ask questions and feel part of the team - part of the process which would help the patient, be it the patient on the table, or the next patient that day, or patients later on in our career. Without this process the surgeons would not have been able to be in the position they were to teach us, and in turn we might be one day to train future students.

A key point in allowing us to feel welcome was the teamwork the surgery team showed for one another and for us as students. The most poignant moment for me was how the surgeon impressed upon us the fact that the patient had consented to this. The patient was also part of a team, the team to train the students.

As much effort as the surgeons had put in to teach us, perhaps it was the patient who had made the ultimate sacrifice. To knowingly allow students to observe and potentially participate, in a controlled environment, in personal surgery is not an easy decision. It is of no benefit to the patient in the short term, and it is understandable that many would not like the idea of strangers being involved at such an intimate level. However, patient consent to students is an indicator of their support of the ideology that this is how students learn to become good doctors and that fundamentally the training process is beneficial and worth the sacrifice. I believe this was a major component in why the surgeons felt able to involve us willingly - the patients consent gave a free and open environment and a positive atmosphere. The patient had the same goals as the surgeon. The patient's consent provided not only an excellent learning tool but helped put the surgeons at ease.

This made me realise why it is so important for the patients to be fully consented for student activities. Not only because of risk and benefit to the patient, but because if the patient has fully informed and is prepared to participate willingly in the educational process for student it enhances and confirms the value of education. In turn, the impact on learning is immense. This has reinforced my appreciation for the patient as part of the educational team, as well as a great sense of humility; that someone who didn't even know me or seen me, was prepared to facilitate my learning. When it comes to learning medicine we are taught that the patient comes first. What is not so obvious is that, during this process, many patients put reservations and fears aside for our medical education to take precedence. This is reflected in the surgeon's attitude towards us and consequently the feeling of teamwork- both educational and medical. I hope I never forget this lesson and that in my future career bring forward this positive attitude of teaching (learnt from the patient) to my students, as the surgeon that day did for us.

COMMENTS ON REFLECTION

This piece mainly concerns the opportunity given to the author of closing up a wound. It highlights the importance of the apprentice system, teamwork and informed consent (although we are not told if the patient gave informed consent for the student to close up). There is mostly descriptive-level reflection in this essay. The majority of the reflective statements from paragraph five onwards are generalisations made about all patients, teams and surgeons rather than about this experience. Reflection is more powerful if it relates to a single patient encounter or event. The author was clearly impressed and felt at ease with the consultant's welcoming approach in theatre but he could have explored here how he felt before and during the suturing. He reflects on consent and the role of patients in general but not in detail about this particular patient. Did the author have any reservations before he sutured? What did he feel during and after the procedure? How did these feelings colour his experience? Did he feel he had done well and did the experience influence what he now wants to do after qualification?

COMMENTS ON ENGLISH
What was done well

➤ This work is methodically and logically laid out and delivered. The student has generally used paragraphs well to separate the stages of the story and thought process, although there is a lone, floating sentence (paragraph five) at the beginning of the reflective section, which should be joined to the following paragraph.

➤ On the whole, the writing style is concise: vocabulary has been deliberately selected to minimise "wordiness" and sentences are generally short and direct. It is important that your essay is easy to follow: long-winded, flowery sentences crammed with inappropriately long words do not impress. A very good essay will seem effortless and should make sense to your reader first time round: maximum meaning will be conveyed through a relatively minimal amount of words. Achieving such succinct and seamless writing is not easy but an exemplary extract from this essay follows, which communicates a lot of meaning in just three sentences:

An issue of much concern had switched to become the best day of learning for me to date. The opportunity I was given by the surgeon, his team and the patient to learn such a valuable practical skill was remarkable, and one which I didn't take for granted. Every student was engaged in some activity that day, but most importantly was encouraged to be involved at some level.

What could have been done better

➤ Although this essay is mostly coherent and straightforward for a reader to follow, there are a few glitches in the writing that probably could have been improved had the student undertaken more thorough proofreading. Many medical students begin their paragraphs in an overly complicated way and hide behind clusters of unnecessary words. It truly is worth taking the extra time to work out how best to construct your sentences. Try reading them aloud and rework them until they make complete sense to you and you are confident that others could also understand them easily. Remember, perfect spoken English is not that different to perfect written English: if it doesn't make sense aloud, it won't make sense on paper. The following examples show how the student has slipped into areas of awkward phrasing, which need to be simplified to be rectified:

Original student version

This has reinforced my appreciation for the patient as part of the educational team, as well as a great sense of humility; that someone who didn't even know me or seen me, was prepared to facilitate my learning.

Amended version

Patients put their trust in the medical team and medical students, who they don't "know" and may not have seen before surgery. Patients are fundamentally important in medical education and I find this humbling.

Original student version

As much effort as the surgeons had put in to teach us, perhaps it was the patient who had made the ultimate sacrifice.

Amended version

The surgeons had put in a lot of effort to teach us but I think the patient's participation and willingness to help us was even more memorable.

In the first week the majority of medical school freshers place orders for stethoscopes, knowing full well that they were up to three years away from needing one for clinical medicine. For three years they were publicly displayed on our shelves or door handles colleting dust, as a reminder of what we were aiming for and to highlight to all potential visitors that we were medical students and proud. Come year three and the first time we are allowed to brush off the cobwebs and wear it round our necks and they become surgically attached to our jugulars, roaming around the hospital basking in the instant recognition we get. Nurses are accustomed to the medical students and identify them by the terror in their eyes as they wander the ward or try to carry out a clinical procedure, but to patients we have the potential to come across as confident clinical practitioners.

However the pride in being instantly recognisable as a medic has its downsides, whether its from friends that grill you about their relative's cancer or ingrown toenail to patients in the lift who try to engage in conversation about their treatment and prognosis. It can be tiring and uncomfortable, as they open up to you in a way you know they wouldn't had you not been instantly recognisable as a medic.

When running into the canteen to grab a coffee in the middle of the day, I momentarily hovered at the sideboard to add milk and sugar and am almost instantly approached by a middle-aged man who asked me whether I was a doctor. I politely reply that I am a medical student and still have 2.5 years to go until I graduate. He immediately launches in to a shining declaration that he thinks doctors are fantastic and the work they do is incredible, and despite the fact that his young daughter had died in intensive care he couldn't praise the staff enough. While previously I had been unengaged, hearing him tell me something that I don't believe he would have said to just anyone standing in the canteen made me turn around and engage, I offered my condolences and he carried on. We ended up sitting down at a table and the conversation went through the recent years of his life; through his daughters death in and the circumstances surrounding it, the breakdown of his marriage, him trying to get revenge for his daughters death and his arrest and finally admission to psychiatric care. I barely said a word during the 90-minute encounter, I didn't need to.

Being quite private person and rarely divulging personal information to even close friends, having a complete stranger talk to me about some of the darkest, most difficult parts of his life made me think about the trust patients put in us from the moment we meet them as medical students/ doctors. Patients will willingly discuss personal details about symptoms and experiences, whether embarrassing, sexual or taboo, with doctors potentially being the only person they have ever divulged the information to. They will undress and expose themselves because they trust that it is both necessary and done in good faith, that they are not being judged and that all information obtained from the encounter will be kept confidential and used to improve their outcome. It is in thinking about this level of trust that led to me really thinking about the qualities of a good doctor for the first time independent of a PDS session or lecture. Maintaining the trust and confidence a patient imparts on a doctor is so important that a god doctor must recognise it, fully appreciate it and build their clinical character and skills around it. Although we have the skills required to make us a good doctor drilled into us from day one at medical school, it wasn't until now that I appreciated why these skills are so important to practice.

It would take just one bad experience with a doctor to break the trust a patient has for their doctors, and even with the most clinically competent doctors working on their case after that their experience and therefore treatment has potentially been compromised. It is important to teach medical students why certain qualities are important and relate them to experiences in their practice, through exercises such as reflective essays, in order for them to appreciate why certain traits and skills are important in clinical practice and the consequences for the patient if they are not upheld.

No matter what area of medicine someone is practising in, different specialities and different levels of care, they are part of one team as far as the patient is concerned with overlapping responsibilities and duties of care and each approached based on the patient's previous clinical experiences.

Medical students, being recognisable as part of the same team, have an equal responsibility to treat the patient with respect and work hard to maintain the trust and confidence patients hold in the medical professionals. A reckless or seemingly uncaring medical student will reflect badly on all other medical students and the medical profession as a whole and appreciating this is critical.

Its not just a stethoscope we are wearing around our necks, it's a siren and should be a constant reminder that we are part of a team and we have the same responsibilities as any doctor. Patients turn to medical professionals to help them through the most difficult times of their lives and we need to appreciate this and give them our full attention, compassion and maintain the highest levels of clinical competence to guarantee the best possible quality of care and outcome for every patient.

COMMENTS ON REFLECTION

This is quite a well-written and well-crafted piece, although the typographical and grammatical errors distract the reader and detract from the enjoyment of reading the essay. It does not have much critical reflection but is rather an opinion piece on medical students' behaviour and attitude. The paragraphs beginning "Being quite private person" and "Its not just a stethoscope we are wearing around our necks" are both moments in the account that are crying out for some detailed reflection (and some proofreading) about the personal meaning of the encounter.

The author touches on a good point: the potentially fragile trust a patient has in their doctor and how this might damage the professional relationship. This issue could have been expanded and would have been a very good subject for reflection, relating the author's perception of what he thinks patients consider fault lines in the doctor–patient relationship and what circumstances and situations might cause an irreparable crack. Breach in confidentiality, lack of informed consent, clinical negligence, persistent rudeness and callous or cold behaviour or simply disinterest are common examples.

COMMENTS ON ENGLISH
What was done well
➤ Parts of this essay are written in a very humorous way and this makes for an entertaining reading experience. Whilst your reflective writing does not need to be humorous (weak jokes are far worse than absent jokes), if you are comfortable with writing in this kind of way it can add a personal dimension to your account. Here is an extract that exemplifies the strength of humour:

Come year three, and the first time we are allowed to brush off the cobwebs and wear it round our necks and they become surgically attached to our jugulars, roaming around the hospital basking in the instant recognition we get. Nurses are accustomed to the medical students and identify them by the terror in their eyes as they wander the ward or try to carry out a clinical procedure, but to patients we have the potential to come across as confident clinical practitioners.

What could have been done better
➤ Whilst parts of this essay are well written, it is let down hugely by its tense inconsistencies, poor punctuation and lack of attention to grammatical detail. The student dithers among the past, present and future tenses in an alarming way and this actually distracts from the event they are trying to relate. The following extract repeatedly flits between the past and present tenses when the whole extract should be either all in the present tense, or, preferably, all in the past tense. Remember, if you are retelling an event that happened in the past, you need to use the past tense.

Original student version
When running into the canteen to grab a coffee in the middle of the day, I momentarily hovered at the sideboard to add milk and sugar and am almost instantly approached by a middle-aged man who asked me whether I was a doctor. I politely reply that I am a medical student and still have 2.5 years to go until I graduate. He immediately launches in to a shining declaration that he thinks doctors are fantastic and the work they do is incredible, and despite the fact that his young daughter had died in intensive care he couldn't praise the staff enough. While previously I had been unengaged, hearing him tell me something that I don't believe he would have said to just anyone standing in the canteen made me turn around and engage, I offered my condolences and he carried on.

Amended version
When I ran into the canteen to grab a coffee in the middle of the day, I momentarily hovered at the sideboard to add milk and sugar and was almost instantly approached by a middle-aged man who asked me whether I was a doctor. I politely replied that I was a medical student and still had two and a half years to go until I graduated. He immediately launched into a shining declaration about how he thought doctors were fantastic and their work was incredible. Despite the fact that his young daughter had died in intensive care, he couldn't praise the staff highly enough. Although initially I found it difficult to believe that he would have disclosed

to a stranger such personal and private emotions, I was happy to talk with him and offered my condolences.

➤ Like all essays, this piece of work would have benefited from thorough proofreading. Typos such as "god doctor" instead of "good doctor" and some overstuffed, poorly constructed sentences (such as, "It would take just one bad experience with a doctor to break the trust a patient has for their doctors, and even with the most clinically competent doctors working on their case after that their experience and therefore treatment has potentially been compromised") are arguably more memorable than the reflection itself. Unfortunately, this sentence highlights the principle that if, when reading your essay aloud, it does not make sense, then it needs to be rewritten and re-punctuated until it reads easily and makes complete sense.

On my Care of the Older Person (COOP) module my group and I went on a home visit to a patient's house as part of our weekly GP placement in Edgeware. The patient we saw was an Indian man of Ugandan origin who had suffered a stroke 6 years ago leaving him with a disability on the right side of his body and an inability to speak and eat. He still had complete mental cognition.

We spoke to the patient and examined him. He was able to understand everything that we were saying but could only respond to us with signs using his able hand, facial expressions and other non-verbal signals. We then spoke to his wife about the situation who was his main carer.

The man himself seemed very depressed and repeatedly expressed wishes to die. He appeared to be very angry with his wife and son for allowing him to live. He had a poor quality of life, staying in bed most of the morning and watching T.V the rest of the day. He only left the house once a week when an external carer took him out for a walk down the street.

His wife explained to us in private that he was a very active man before the stroke, extremely sociable and talkative. She thought the worst repercussions of the stroke for him were the inability to talk and the inability to eat- apparently he used to love going to eat out at different restaurants with friends. The wife said she herself was getting used to communicating with him without words but his anger towards her and the change in his personality were the hardest things to deal with. She said the man sitting in the room next door was completely unrecognisable as the man that she married 45 years ago.

I felt very sorry for the man himself and perhaps more so for his family who had to look after him and stay emotionally strong for him. The wife was depressed and hardly left the house herself. His son had a burden of responsibilities upon his shoulders, not being only the main breadwinner of the family but also the only person who could speak fluent English. He therefore had the responsibility of arranging all hospital appointments, carers, bills etc. I felt sad because the atmosphere in the house was stiflingly depressing and hopeless. I felt sorry for the patient and his family because I could leave and get back to my normal life after the home visit whereas they could not escape the situation. The issue of euthanasia had also crossed my thoughts, and whether it should be an option for patients in situations like this (although my personal moral and religious beliefs, after much deliberation, did lead me to conclude that euthanasia should not be legalised in Britain).

The outcome of the experience for me was that it gave me an insight into the lives of patients outside the hospital environment. I actually saw and appreciated the hardships that go on at home, that we as hospital students/doctors often do not think about deeply enough. The outcome for the patient and the family was that they were able to communicate with some new fresh faces which I think they enjoyed.

I believe the experience was very good for me and my future working as a doctor. It gave me a greater insight into the lives of patients and seeing them at home made me really wonder how I would feel if this was someone in my own family, rather than feeling emotionally detached from the situation as I sometimes do during clerking in hospital (especially during the Surgery module). I believe that my own actions during both consultations (with husband and wife) were considerate, compassionate and professional. The experience also enhanced my abilities in communicating effectively with patients who are unable to speak, and I believe that I managed to get a lot of information out of him considering the circumstances.

In the future will always consider how the patient and their family are able to cope with an illness/injury outside hospital. I will always ask if they have enough home help and bear in mind that antidepressants or counselling may be an important option for many patients. I will also always think about the financial repercussions that may arise from serious illness.

COMMENTS ON REFLECTION

This is a good reflective essay and includes all the required components. What is particularly good is that the author has chosen as her topic the very difficult issue of euthanasia and has tried to analyse her own reactions to the situation rather than offer an opinion.

As a professional learning experience, she identified with the patient and the family and learned that medical care and problems exist out of hospital and are at least as difficult to manage in the patient's home. The experience seems to have taught her about the practical and financial consequences of chronic disease.

There are still areas where this piece could be improved. The description is full and could be shortened. The author asserts that her actions "during both consultations (with husband and wife) were considerate, compassionate and professional" but she does not provide evidence for why she thinks this is the case.

COMMENTS ON ENGLISH

What was done well

➤ The student generally uses short, simple sentences that effectively describe a complex situation. This essay is void of the flowery language that many medical students employ and the result is good: clear thoughts and feelings articulated in a concise way. Whilst some sentences are syntactically problematic, they are effectively worded and are mostly of an appropriate length.

What could have been done better

➤ The general quality of the writing is not bad but it is let down by spelling and grammatical errors. It is imperative that key spellings, including the names of hospitals and placements, are correct. Spelling words such as "Edgware" incorrectly (the student spells it "Edgeware") makes the writer look sloppy and inattentive, particularly as she went to the hospital on several occasions, saw the hospital sign and the hospital signage and notepaper.

➤ Some of the sentences are structured in a confusing way, hindering the clarity and meaning of the writing. The phrase "We then spoke to his wife about the situation who was his main carer" is badly ordered. It reads as if the situation was his main carer. A clearer and more accurate version of the sentence could read: "We then spoke to his wife, his main carer, about the situation." This reordered sentence, which uses bracketing commas to divide the clauses (a clause is a fragment of a sentence which can be removed to leave a grammatically complete sentence), clearly shows that the subject, his wife, was the main carer.

When looking back at my first term as a clinical medical student, one incident always springs to mind. It was at the very start of the term and I was rushing to get to a colorectal clinic. As I arrived I could see a nurse pushing a gentleman in a wheelchair into the room. She was struggling greatly and I offered to help her. Even with my help, it was very difficult to push the man and we had to seek further help from another medical student.

The gentleman could barely fit into the wheelchair due to his size. In addition, he was holding his legs up with a piece of material so that they would not drag onto the floor. I had never seen a gentleman so large – I was quite shocked at the sight. Once we finally got him into the room with the help of the Doctor, the consultation began. I found I was actually observing a bariatric clinic, which for me was a great eye opening and thought provoking experience.

The patient was a 35 year old Caucasian male and he had a BMI of around 44. I had barely sat down and taken a pen out when I heard the surgeon abruptly say 'Sorry Sir but due to your heart conditions we do not think you are suitable to have a general anaesthetic and therefore we will be unable to offer you a gastric bypass'. There was silence in the room. The man didn't seem surprised. He just looked down and handed the Doctor a bag so that he could make sure all his medications were fine.
I was rather perplexed. What were the alternatives? What other options did he have? This man was still very young, he clearly had serious problems and he needed help!

As we managed to dismiss the patient with great difficulty (the wheelchair was hard to push and required around 3 people) I sat with the Doctor and asked him what would happen now. It seemed as though this happened everyday. The Doctor did not look alarmed or worried in any way, but was simply filling out some forms. We sat back down and I waited for him to finish. He then looked up and said to me 'the patient has heart conditions, sleep apnoea; it is unlikely he will live for much longer'. And that was it! The clinic was actually over.

I walked slowly back to the common room. I kept going over what had happened in my head. I felt a little sad inside. Surely it can't be his fault that he is obese. There may be genetic factors involved or their may have been an episode in his life that led him to eat excessively. He could have even gone through some depression or something. Maybe he'd had some leg or back surgery that prevented him from exercising or moving around. I kept thinking he was not to blame. He looked so defeated when he was told the shocking news. I felt really sorry for him and felt really helpless myself.

When I got back, everyone could tell I looked a little upset. One of my colleagues asked me what was wrong and I told him what I had observed. He had a completely different opinion compared to me. He said that it was entirely the gentleman's fault and that he should have watched what he ate and had self-control. My colleague believed that the patient should have realised what was happening and done something about it. I was so confused. I didn't know what to think. I tried to defend the gentleman saying maybe something had forced him to eat excessively and that their may have been personal reasons but no matter what I said, he was not convinced. He believed that the gentleman himself was to blame for his condition.

Three months have passed since the incident, yet I still cannot forget what has happened. Before that day, I knew what obesity was, I knew it was a growing problem in the west, yet I hadn't fully understood how it affected people's lives. Now I don't know what to think anymore. I want to help these people. There must be a way in which obese people can be helped. It is not fair that they leave this world at such a young age – but then I cannot help thinking, is what my colleague said right? Are they really to blame? Even if the gentleman was to blame, everyone makes mistakes and I am certain the man would do anything for a second chance.

COMMENTS ON REFLECTION

The author has written compellingly, describing his frustration and sadness about the patient and how he remained upset about the patient's future, three months after the incident. During the intervening three months, the author has not appeared to use this memorable clinical event to learn about the condition and how he would cope emotionally and practically if he were to encounter other obese patients. Reflecting on our emotions is only the first stage of reflective practice. We need to move on and explore the episode from a number of perspectives; to mull things over with the aim of leading to a greater understanding and improved patient care. The author missed the opportunity to reflect on the doctor's statement that the patient would be "unlikely to live for long", and he did not question the doctor about this. He also did not explore the dissonance of his views and the apparent views of others. The essay is thus mainly descriptive and, whilst it does have some superficial reflection, the author has not completed the reflective process.

COMMENTS ON ENGLISH

What was done well

➤ This essay is written in a lively style that is characterised with a great variety of sentence structures and lengths. A blend of rhetorical questions, long sentences, shorter sentences and even a few exclamation marks make for interesting reading and enliven the account. It is worth considering such grammatical and structural detail when writing, as the quality of your expression can truly add a lot to your account. An extract that is particularly strong for these reasons is: "There was silence in the room. The man didn't seem surprised. He just looked down and handed the Doctor a bag so that he could make sure all his medications were fine.

I was rather perplexed. What were the alternatives? What other options did he have? This man was still very young, he clearly had serious problems and he needed help!"

What could have been done better

➤ There is not one major problem area in this piece of work but the essay is peppered with minor grammatical glitches that detract from our overall impression of the piece of work. The student begins some sentences with the word "and", which is usually frowned upon as "and" is a connective, used to join, not begin, sentences. The student also refers to "the west", which implies a general westerly direction, but the student should have capitalised "the West" as they were actually referring to a specific area, which is a proper noun requiring an upper-case W. The student has also used dashes where colons, commas or semicolons would have sufficed. Dashes are informal and are not appropriate for academic pieces of writing.

CHAPTER 4

Self-assessment exercises

INTRODUCTION

You have now read a wide range of reflective essays that illustrate both satisfactory and unsatisfactory reflective practice. You should now have a clear understanding of what constitutes good reflective writing, the problems that commonly arise in terms of both content and style and how to improve your written English.

Whether you are an author developing your self-critiquing skills or a reflective practice teacher who needs to give feedback to learners, you should use these final five pieces as an opportunity to test yourself. Each of these final five essays is followed by a blank page for you to write down your comments on the reflection and written English. We then provide our comments as a guide. Read the pieces carefully; identify their strengths and weaknesses and the ways in which they could be improved.

We would like to remind you that we do not consider our views as the only "correct" way to comment on reflective essays. Throughout this book, we have tried to emphasise the fundamentals of reflective practice and good English. We hope this book has been helpful and that these final self-assessment exercises will consolidate your own reflection.

One of the difficulties with the General Medical Specialities rotation is trying to gain exposure to each of the different specialities while you are attached to a single firm for the duration of the block. Having had a few weeks of settling into Haematology I decided it was time to make a start on trying to get to grips with Endocrinology and so I went along to a general endocrine clinic. I asked the consultant running the clinic if he would mind me sitting in on his consultations. He was initially extremely accommodating and in fact set me up in a side room of my own to clerk patients and subsequently present my findings to him. The first consultation ran smoothly and he seemed pleased with my history and examination findings. The second case, however, proved to be a lot more difficult for reasons which I could not have anticipated. During the second consultation, in which I was already feeling out of my depth because I had to communicate with a non-English speaking patient via an interpreter, a different doctor opened the door to my side room without knocking and asked me sharply, 'Why did you not attend the lecture this morning?' This took me by complete surprise as I was totally unaware of any lecture I was supposed to be attending that morning. The doctor proceeded to scold me, in front of the patient and the interpreter, suggesting that I had made a conscious decision against going to the lecture which she had organised. She knew this because a student from the endocrine firm had arrived at the clinic after the lecture. The door was then closed only to be opened again two minutes later by the consultant who remarked, 'I believe you are not one of our own, you will have to leave and let this student take over from you because she is supposed to be here and you are not'. The consultant then directed the student into my consultation room and closed the door. Essentially what had started out as a professional interview between the patient, the interpreter and me became a farce. I was left feeling embarrassed, shocked and upset at being spoken to in front of a fellow student and a patient in such a way. How could the patient have maintained any kind of respect for me as a future doctor having just witnessed this outburst? I did my best to remain professional and continue the interview but within minutes the consultant re-entered the room and asked me to present my findings to him. He must have known that because of the interruptions I would not have been able to conduct the interview properly and to the best of my ability yet he still told me that my effort was pathetic and sarcastically said 'I think your time would have been better spent attending the lecture this morning, don't you?' I was mortified and fighting back tears throughout the remainder of the consultation whilst my fellow student kept looking over at me trying to signal that she was sorry for getting me into trouble. When the consultation was over, I collected my belongings and swiftly left the room thinking, 'Did that really just happen?' I burst into tears. I had genuinely not known about the lecture otherwise I would have been there. All that I had been trying to do was take initiative and further my education. I wanted desperately to go back and explain to the consultant that there had been a misunderstanding but I felt that it would do no good. He had already made his mind up about me and made it very clear what he thought about the situation. The rest of the day I spent ruminating on what had happened that morning, playing the events over and over in my head. It emerged that there had been an administrative error and my haematology firm had not received the email detailing the lectures scheduled for Thursday mornings. As the day went on, my tears turned to anger. I am still shocked at how rude the consultant was to me. What angered me most was that he didn't even give me the chance to explain. I later found out that he has upset other students before. In retrospect I should have been stronger and reported this situation to a more senior figure but I couldn't help but feel at the time that it would do no good. After all, he is a consultant and I am a mere student. It will be important for me in the coming years to develop a more effective way of handling disputes between myself and other members of the team. Since that day I have avoided returning to the endocrine department, probably because I associate the place with how I felt on that day- humiliated, upset and angry. I realise now that he had no right to make me feel this way and in the future I would most definitely act upon it for my own sake but also for the sake of my fellow students.

PLEASE COMMENT ON THE REFLECTIVE AND ENGLISH COMPONENTS OF THIS ESSAY:

COMMENTS ON REFLECTION

This piece describes vividly the author's emotional upset in clinic following missing a lecture. She felt humiliated, hurt, embarrassed, frustrated, out of her depth and angry after a doctor reprimanded her in front of a non-English-speaking patient for missing a lecture. The consultant running the clinic then made a comment that caused her further upset.

Instead of taking a step back and exploring her reactions, and the possible reasons for her upset with the two doctors, most of her essay is a long explanation or justification for why she felt the way she did and a complaint about the way she was treated. Reflection is designed to allow the writer to express how they felt and describe their emotions, but this should lead to a more analytical and objective assessment of why they felt the way they did, what they learned from the experience and what they would do if a similar event occurred again.

The author ruminates on her experience, tells the reader about the administrative mistake with the lecture and describes her residual anger with the consultant who "didn't even give me the chance to explain". She could have explored possible solutions, for example speaking to the consultant, who would probably have listened to her and apologised for any upset he caused. She concludes, correctly, that she will have to toughen up in order to survive the interpersonal jousting that is part and parcel of clinical life and also part of most workplace interactions. It will not be long before she will be in a senior position and this experience will have been of help to her.

What would have made this a much better reflective piece would have been a more objective exploration of why she felt the way she did at the time, what she learned from a rather unpleasant experience, how she would deal with a similar predicament next time and whether, ironically, she thinks she learned more from this event than from the lecture she missed.

Students and doctors must learn from all events, particularly the emotionally traumatic ones. You have to be able to "let things go", so that you retain your sanity and good humour, and reflecting purposefully on experiences like this helps with that process.

The only mention of the patient here, who may have been feeling equally uncomfortable, is in relation to the author: how she was made to look unprofessional and how unpleasant the experience was for her. Perhaps this was also something to explore.

COMMENTS ON ENGLISH

What was done well

➤ This piece of work is generally written in a clear and detailed style. The student has carefully considered the event in a logical way and the reader finds it easy to follow the events described. When writing reflectively it is key that you include detail in an interesting and relevant way. A good way of enlivening your account is varying sentence structure and length as this varies the pace of your writing. Another good way to make your writing exciting is to be adventurous with your vocabulary choices. The following extract is a good example of how the student has used speech, rhetorical questions and original expression:

Essentially what had started out as a professional interview between the patient, the interpreter and me became a farce. I was left feeling embarrassed, shocked and upset at being spoken to in front of a fellow student and a patient in such a way. How could the patient have maintained any kind of respect for me as a future doctor having just witnessed this outburst? I did my best to remain professional and continue the interview but within minutes the consultant re-entered the room and asked me to present my findings to him.

What could have been done better

➤ This essay is not divided into paragraphs and reads as one big "lump" of essay. This makes the work intimidating and difficult for a reader to approach. Your essay plan should, ideally, involve you considering your work in terms of paragraphs and if, upon completing your work, you find your essay paragraph-less you may need to review it carefully and segment your writing. Whilst transitions from paragraph to paragraph should be grammatically and thematically seamless, paragraph breaks should follow shifts in time, action or thought. For example, the first paragraph break could separate the first consultation from the second consultation:

Original student version

The second case, however, proved to be a lot more difficult for reasons which I could not have anticipated. During the second consultation, in which I was already feeling out of my depth because I had to communicate with a non-English speaking patient via an interpreter, a different doctor entered the clinic room opened the door to my side room without knocking and asked me sharply, 'Why did you not attend the lecture this morning?'

Amended version

The second case, however, proved to be a lot more difficult, for reasons I could not have anticipated.

During the second consultation, in which I was already feeling out of my depth because I had to communicate with a non-English-speaking patient via an interpreter, a different doctor opened the door to my side room without knocking and asked me sharply, 'Why did you not attend the lecture this morning?'

From the two days spend on Critical Care I have reflected upon the importance of confidence, competence and professionalism. Two events that stood out to me were practising the DRABCDE in the clinical skills lab and carrying out DRABCDE is practice by the bedside of a critically ill patient.

Due to recent events I have found myself to be deflated and less confident in groups, which used to be my forte. I was enthusiastic around the clock and some may say hyperactive when is comes to getting stuck in to practical activities, suggesting clinics would be a dream.

During the DRABCDE in clinical skills the effects of life events on me became apparent. I realised that it was affecting me more than I thought. I was unable to let go and just go for it; instead I was quiet, uncomfortable and unconfident. After I saw other students carry out the DRABCDE after me, I realised the importance of acting confident, speaking clearly and not hesitating and primarily just saying what you think confidently. I did not feel frustrated or unhappy, it was more a realisation of what I need to do to improve myself and my clinically based learning –which I feel I learn better from as opposed to sitting quietly in a minimally interactive lecture.

When we carried out the DRABCDE by the bedside and generally in clinical practice, I realised the importance of being a professional being for the patients sake. I felt that if you were confident, this instils trust in the patient and makes them more comfortable with you for example taking their blood or cannulating. I also observed that as medical students and future doctors, we need to be aware of the effects of confidence in a position of authority on patients. This was apparent when we asked the patient's permission to feel her pulse and she replied "whatever you need to do" and our clinical skills tutor reinforced to the patient that she doesn't have to let us do anything she doesn't want to. It is remarkable how much trust and power patients give doctors/ medical student with their care –a privilege not to be abused or forgotten. I must not forget throughout my career to remind patients of their choice and free will. However, I also came to understand the importance of practising DRABCDE assessments, taking histories, clinical examinations, taking blood etc. on patients that may not reap any benefit from it or presenting to doctors that will already know the whole history. I need to practice so that I am able to carry out these skills confidently as a doctor and so I need to get over the uncomfortable feeling of being a pest or asking personal questions. I now understand that it may not benefit this particular patient, but it will benefit others (obviously, if the patient has consented). At the same time, I observed how some steps in the DRABCDE assessment of the patient were omitted in order to avoid distressing the patient unnecessarily, for example, asking the patient to sit up and listen to her lungs posteriorly.

On a more positive side note, recent events have given me real life experience and I feel that I am more equip to understand patients' emotions.

To summarise, from my experience during critical care, I have realised that my action points are to be more confident and comfortable for the benefit of myself and the patient, and, to constantly remind myself of the ease of patient coercion and to avoid this by reminding the patient of their autonomy throughout my career.

PLEASE COMMENT ON THE REFLECTIVE AND ENGLISH COMPONENTS OF THIS ESSAY:

COMMENTS ON REFLECTION

This is a first attempt at reflective practice by this author and it shows in a number of ways. Often reflective writing is treated by novices as a "stream of consciousness"; a little like what one might write in a personal diary. If one decides to approach reflective writing in this way the resulting written piece should be treated as a very rough first draft rather than the piece for submission. Here there is lack of clarity about exactly what is being reflected upon: is it about how life events affect practice? Is it about confidence? Practice? Consent? The veiled reference to life events in the third paragraph seems to assume the reader knows what those life events were. Together with the constantly changing tense and the lack of proofreading (which unfortunately results in a mistake as early as the first sentence), this piece actually gives the impression of someone who cannot take the time to reflect purposefully and cannot spare the time to proofread. The great author Samuel Johnson wrote: "What is written without effort is in general read without pleasure". If this piece of reflective practice was being used for "proof" of reflective growth or, indeed, for selection or appraisal, this piece is in fact rather counterproductive.

COMMENTS ON ENGLISH
What was done well

➤ This essay is generally written in a concise and direct style. Although there are a few clichés, this essay does not suffer from the "wordiness" that flaws some pieces of reflective writing. Most of the sentences make sense upon their first reading and the incident described is, therefore, relatively easy for a reader to follow.

What could have been done better

➤ Parts of this work demonstrate the pitfalls of a computer spellcheck. Whilst your computer will never supply you with an incorrectly spelled option, it can often supply you with the wrong word altogether. This student has, unfortunately, included such a typo in her opening paragraphs and, whilst the mistake seems minor, it detracts from the overall quality of her work and indicates sloppiness:

Original student version

Two events that stood out to me were practising the DRABCDE in the clinical skills lab and carrying out DRABCDE is practice by the bedside of a critically ill patient.

Amended version

Two events that stood out to me were practising the DRABCDE in the clinical skills lab and carrying out DRABCDE in practice by the bedside of a critically ill patient. [Not all readers will know what DRABCDE stands for and this should have been written in full (Danger, Response, Airway, Breathing, Circulation, Defibrillation, Environment).]

➤ The student has included a few clichés in their work, which is a shame. Whilst clichés are easily absorbed in everyday spoken English, they should be avoided at all costs in formal pieces of academic writing. Clichés are, by definition, overused phrases that are, by default, meaningless and bland. They are also far too informal and colloquial for reflective writing and will not help you convey the specifics of the situation you are reflecting on as they are quite generic and vague.

Original student version
I was enthusiastic around the clock and some may say hyperactive when is comes to getting stuck in to practical activities, suggesting clinics would be a dream.

Amended version
I had always been enthusiastic about practical activities and so I looked forward to working in clinic.

Original student version
I was unable to let go and just go for it.

Amended version
I was unable to relax and engage comfortably with the patients.

➤ This essay is well paragraphed to a point, but towards the end the student decides to finish with two bizarrely isolated sentences that should be joined together and possibly to another paragraph. A paragraph should generally be at least three sentences long.

In my essay on reflective practice, I have decided to reflect upon an incident that occurred during the module gone by, that of Care of the Elderly; I feel that in the context of this module, and indeed of modern medicine in general, the incident I am bringing up is particularly appropriate reflecting a difficult issue that, in my opinion, must cross the paths of all practising doctors, if not then at least all doctors responsible for the teaching of students. While I was not specifically involved and only watched the incident unfold, it nevertheless made a profound and lasting impact on me.

The incident occurred during a GP placement I was attached to, for which we visited a hospice one week to examine some local patients of the surgery. Having obtained consent from the patients the previous day, our GP asked the carers to bring them to us. The first patient that was brought to us was a middle aged woman, around 40 years of age, who clearly had Down's syndrome from her appearance. At first, the patient seemed amicable enough, and was brought by a carer into one of the rooms; the GP, the other students and I followed them in. There were two boys and two girls in our group and in this instance our GP had decided to split us up into pairs, both girls together and both boys together. The girls were to examine this first patient and approached the patient and the carer on the other side of the room. As they did so, the patient seemed to be getting uncomfortable, and the two girls hesitated. I mentioned that perhaps the patient was claustrophobic and that us two boys and the GP should leave the room, but the GP wanted to make sure the girls were ok before departing. As the girls got closer the patient started to cry, at which point the girls appeared to be unsure what to do. However, the carer calmed the patient down and informed her that the girls were just going to listen to her chest and then she would be able to go back to what she was doing. For a while the patient seemed less distressed but as the girls moved to expose her chest the patient once more became very distressed and started crying again, clearly uncomfortable with the situation. The GP, addressing the carer at this point, said that it was ok and we could come back another time or examine another patient. However, the carer repeatedly ensured both the GP and the girls that once the patient realised that all the girls were doing was a respiratory examination she would calm down and be fine once more. The GP, still looking unsure, told the girls to go ahead and perform the examination. At this point the GP and my pair left to find our own patient. However, I later learned that when the girls tried to examine the patient, she wouldn't stop crying, and were unsure what to do. The carer exposed the chest and the girls performed a quick superficial examination and concluded, thanking the patient; when I spoke to them, the girls seemed agitated about the experience, unsure whether they should have even performed it at all.

When I was in that patient's room, I think I thought that as the GP knew the patient personally and had obtained consent the day before, he and the carer would be best at judging whether it was ok to go ahead with the examination. I have found in the past months of ward work that a similar situation, where the patient is a bit hesitant at giving consent but the doctor reassures you and tells you to go ahead with the examination, is quite common, especially in an environment where students are required to perform supervised examinations and the doctors are required to allow students to 'learn by doing' on a daily basis. In terms of the incident at the care home, the consequences to the patient were that they were made to feel uncomfortable for a period of about 10 minutes, indeed the same can be said of the students involved. The issue here, in my opinion is whether the examination should have gone on at all. Were the previous consent and the assurances of the patient's carer enough? Or should the GP have told the students not to perform the examination?

The relevant information from the GMC guidelines state that performing an examination of any sort on a patient that has not provided consent, with full mental capacity and informed knowledge of the outcomes, is battery and against the law. However, the issue here is clouded by the fact that the patient was informed as she had been examined by students before and it was assumed by the GP, that she had full mental capacity to make that decision. However, the patient seemed uncomfortable at the point of examination while not explicitly saying that she withdrew her consent. Obviously had she said this, the examination would not have gone ahead; if the carer or even the GP hadn't intervened I think the students certainly would have and would have declined to perform the examination. Nevertheless, the GP was unsure about the course of action as the reason she was crying was not entirely clear. With hindsight, to be safe the GP should have decided it perhaps wasn't absolutely necessary and the girls could have found another patient, but in his mind he perhaps knew that given the respiratory signs that this patient had, another patient might not be such a good learning experience. In addition the girls, in my opinion, shouldn't have performed the examination when the patient started to cry again upon trying to expose her, and should have perhaps talked to the patient more beforehand. If the patient was still distressed I think they should have left the room and informed the GP.

Normally, patients do not get this distressed, but I think if I see this in future I will know better how to deal with the patient. It would have been helpful to the GP I think if my pair, as a 3rd party, had spoken up to say that it was best not to examine the patient while she was feeling like that. And that the girls could have examined our own, the second, patient who turned out to be a pleasant elderly woman. I'm glad the incident has occurred early in my medical career as I can now learn from it and support others where they are unsure about the course of action.

**PLEASE COMMENT ON THE REFLECTIVE AND ENGLISH
COMPONENTS OF THIS ESSAY:**

COMMENTS ON REFLECTION

"In my essay on reflective practice" is not a promising start. The point of reflective writing is not to write about reflection or about something or someone but about a personally important incident. The first paragraph is not necessary and does not help us to understand the author or the situation. The next descriptive paragraph is also overlong. The main flaw with this piece is that it involves the author as a bystander, making judgements and assumptions regarding the intentions and actions of others. Criticism is levelled at the carer, the GP and the other students; was she not in any way complicit as a silent bystander?

The sentence where the distress of the patient is reduced to "they were made to feel uncomfortable for a period of about 10 minutes" is very unfortunate. This student now seems to be critical of others, non-reflective of self and uncaring towards patients! It is worth rereading written pieces like this with fresh eyes (as if you had not been there) to explore for unintended meanings and ensure you as the author are at the heart of the experience.

COMMENTS ON ENGLISH

What was done well

➤ There is some attempt to vary the structure of some sentences here, making for interesting reading: no one enjoys reading an essay where all the sentences begin in the same way.

➤ A particularly effective part of the essay features rhetorical questions that are thought-provoking and exciting: "The issue here, in my opinion is whether the examination should have gone on at all. Were the previous consent and the assurances of the patient's carer enough? Or should the GP have told the students not to perform the examination?" A lot of students do include rhetorical questions in their writing and they are generally good additions to make as they indicate a deeper train of thought and an understanding of the complexity of the situation.

What could have been done better

➤ The main grammatical weaknesses of this essay lies in its syntax. The essay is wordy, slightly rambling and also incoherent at times as sentences are poorly constructed and "overstuffed". The opening sentence is particularly weak because you should try to make your introductions and conclusions very strong to create a favourable impression on your reader. The improved version, which follows, has addressed the main grammatical issues: sentence length, sentence structure, unnecessary words and repetition of key ideas. Good writing is concise and precise; every word should matter. Note how the improved version is about half the length of the student version yet retains all meaning:

Original student version

In my essay on reflective practice, I have decided to reflect upon an incident that occurred during the module gone by, that of Care of the Elderly; I feel that in the context of this module, and indeed of modern medicine in general, the incident I am bringing up is particularly appropriate reflecting a difficult issue that, in my opinion, must cross the paths of all practising doctors, if not then at least all doctors responsible for the teaching of students.

Amended version

I have decided to reflect upon an incident that occurred during a previous module in my Care of the Elderly firm attachment. The incident concerned presents a difficult issue that most doctors probably encounter.

➤ The student's levels of formality slip at times: the word "ok" should not enter formal academic writing. First, the student has not capitalised "OK", which is, second, too informal and vague for a reflective piece. Better versions could be "alright", "stable" or "content". Whilst you may tell a colleague on a ward round that a patient is "OK" you should never write the abbreviation in formal writing: good spoken and written English are not always identical. The student has also abbreviated the words "3rd party". Unless quoting a number that is 10 or over, always write the number in letters (this is, "third party").

It was a Monday morning and I had been asked to take an observed history for a bedside teaching session with my firm. The patient was a pleasant forty-year-old Caucasian gentleman on the acute ward, who had been brought in by ambulance following a seizure on his way home from a football match the previous day. This was followed by a second seizure whilst in A&E, which brought him to a total of five seizures in the last seven to eight years. The patient had no history of seizures prior to the last eight years and there was no family history of epilepsy. His only past medical history was oesophageal achalasia and several fractures sustained whilst playing football.

However, the patient commented that these seizures had occurred as 3 separate episodes, each of which was preceded by heavy alcohol consumption. He admitted to being "somewhat of a binge drinker", going to the pub only once a fortnight on average but drinking around 35 units of beer and spirits in one evening. However, he denied any recreational drug use and was not taking any medications.

Once I had presented the history, the predictable discussion of differential diagnoses ensued and the consultant prompted my colleagues to ask all of the relevant questions that I had missed. The consultant felt that these seizures were most likely to be idiopathic but also suggested that they could be the result of hepatotoxicity from the alcohol. She then proceeded to ask myself and my colleagues about the consequences of high alcohol consumption. The patient listened intently to these, and whilst he had already stated his intention to cut down drinking, hearing about these possible outcomes only seemed to add to his resolve.

However, as one of my colleagues went on to examine the patient, the consultant continued to labour the issue of alcohol consumption. She went into great depth about palpating cirrhotic livers and had my colleague scouring the patient's chest for spider naive, until several small ones were located. The patient seemed visibly uncomfortable by this point, as the consultant was using phrases such as 'heavy drinkers' and 'alcoholics' when describing the signs she was asking us to look for. Whilst we as medical students needed to be taught the peripheral stigmata of liver disease, there didn't seem to be the need to direct these comments towards the patient with such zeal. Several times he tried to reassure the consultant that drinking alcohol really wasn't taking over his life as she seemed to be implying with her line of questioning but the consultant dismissed this with an air of scepticism. My peers and I felt quite embarrassed at the lack of tact from the consultant, particularly when she prompted us to enquire more about the fractures he had sustained in case they were due to his falling whilst drunk.

Once we had finished the examination and thanked the patient, we continued down the ward. At this point the consultant admitted that she had pressed the issue of alcohol in order scare the patient into giving up. "In cases like these you've got to," she said. I didn't really have a response at this point. This was a doctor I very much respected and admired for her thorough patient care and I did agree that a patient should know the consequences of lifestyle choices in order that they can make an informed decision. However, I could not condone the kind of verbal bullying which I had witnessed. It was one thing to be firm in one's advice and to enquire about whether alcohol was having an impact on this gentleman's job or family life (which they were not) but quite another to make the patient feel shame and fear, and to make him think that we were expecting to see signs of severe liver disease when the history was really not consistent with this.

Myself and my colleagues were left feeling very sorry for the patient, not because he had received inadequate care but because he had received poor communication of the facts and been made to feel ashamed. In the long term, perhaps this consultant's emphasis on the harmful effects of alcohol was effective in convincing the patient to reduce his intake or even abstain but does this warrant jeopardising the doctor-patient relationship? On his next visit to hospital, will the patient be less likely to participate in student teaching for fear of further embarrassment? Ultimately, one might think that it is worth sacrificing these things for the possibility of extra years added to the patient's life but as doctors we are taught to maintain patient dignity as a foremost concern, and this is something I think we need to be unwilling to sacrifice.

Also, the consultant was merely teaching a group of students, this was not her patient and she probably never saw him again, so there was no opportunity for him to discuss this issue further. This makes him less likely to be able to convert his feelings of embarrassment and worry into a positive change by decreasing his alcohol consumption to safe levels.

Whether this incident had any effect on the patient's physical or mental well-being I will never know, but it has certainly educated me on how to inform patients and make recommendations to aid their health without causing them unnecessary anxiety or upset. It has also taught me that no matter how good a consultant's communication skills, they can still make mistakes and may not handle all situations well. As for the consultant, she obviously did not pick up on the emotional cues of this patient, as a similar situation occurred again several weeks later. In future, I think I might be inclined to tactfully give feedback to doctors, whatever their career stage, and ask about their communication style. In doing so I may be likely to face hostility but providing I am polite and respectful, I may be able to contribute to the personal development of doctors and the healthcare experiences of patients.

PLEASE COMMENT ON THE REFLECTIVE AND ENGLISH COMPONENTS OF THIS ESSAY:

COMMENTS ON REFLECTION

There is a lot of description and very little direct personal reflection here, which is a pity because the author wrote well and sensitively but did not tell us how she felt, why, or how she would have communicated with this patient.

Nearly the whole essay is a recapitulation of her case history and the rest, a critical commentary of what she perceived as poor communication skills and a "bullying" approach by the consultant. She describes the clinical history very well, and we are able to sense the way the teaching went. From a bedside teaching and patient education perspective, it would be appropriate to teach students on alcohol abuse management in relation to this patient. It is impossible for the reader to make a judgement on whether the consultant was "bullying" the patient or being direct about the risks of his binge drinking. If the patient understood the dangers of his binge drinking and did not take offence with the way the consultant spoke to him, then it could be argued that the consultant's communication style was effective.

The author does not tell us what she learned about communication skills, how she would have spoken to the patient, how she would in future discuss alcohol consumption with a patient or how she thinks this important and common medical and social problem should be taught at the bedside. It will not be long before the author may want to teach on the medical complications of alcohol herself. How would she do it at the bedside?

COMMENTS ON ENGLISH
What was done well

➤ The general quality of the English in this essay is good. Whilst it is slightly "wordy", the work is quite easy to follow and the range of vocabulary used combined with the structure of the sentences and paragraphs make for interesting reading. Although this level of writing is acceptable, the student should try to be more economical with her words and consider whether all the words she uses truly add to the meaning she is trying to convey. We can follow the thought process underpinning this essay but, arguably, the word count could have been drastically reduced had some mindful word culling taken place during the proofreading stages.

What could have been done better

➤ This student's grammar is not bad but she has made a very common error involving pronoun and syntax confusion that needs to be addressed:

Original student version
She then proceeded to ask myself and my colleagues about the consequences of high alcohol consumption.

Amended version

She then proceeded to ask me and my colleagues about the consequences of high alcohol consumption.

In this example the student erroneously wrote "myself" instead of "me". Whilst it is tempting to disregard the pronoun "me", you have to consider how the sentence would run without the extra people in it; this is, "She then proceeded to ask myself ~~and my colleagues~~ about the consequences of high alcohol consumption" does not make sense.

The student repeated this mistake further on in the essay:

Original student version

Myself and my colleagues were left feeling very sorry for the patient, not because he had received inadequate care but because he had received poor communication of the facts and been made to feel ashamed.

Amended version

My colleagues and I were left feeling very sorry for the patient, not because he had received inadequate care but because he had received poor communication of the facts and been made to feel ashamed.

In this example the student also erroneously wrote "myself and my colleagues", yet if you take the colleagues out of the sentence ("Myself ~~and my colleagues~~ were left feeling very sorry for the patient . . .") it does not make sense. If you are unsure about which pronoun to use try removing the extra "people" in the sentence and see if the sentence makes sense.

Clinical medicine has been challenging yet exciting. Casting my thoughts back to the introductory course, there was a session on history taking led by a team of PALS tutors (peer-assisted learning). We were already taught the structure of a history, and this session was based on practical clinical scenarios. I was really looking forward to this session because I knew how important history taking skills were and I also wanted to check how much I had retained from the previous session. I wanted to use this as an opportunity to prepare myself for clerking on the wards which was gradually approaching.

In our small group there was a PALS tutor and Mr X who acted out the role of the patient. As always, the PALS tutor tried to make the atmosphere as relaxed as possible and encouraged us to ask questions. Despite knowing this was a learning experience, I still found it difficult to control my nerves and it did not help being the first one up. We were each given a scenario which involved concentrating on a particular aspect of the history for five minutes. My scenario was a gentleman presenting to the GP with abdominal pain and I had to take a detailed history of the presenting complaint.

At the end of the case, I was asked to comment on my own performance beginning with the positives. It is difficult to compliment yourself; I have always found it much easier to criticise myself. Reflecting on the short five minute consultation, I thought I addressed the patient well at the start, explaining the issues of confidentiality. I managed to gather most of the relevant information and summarised it back to the patient to ensure that it was correct and nothing important was omitted. On the contrary, I thought I was quite hesitant at asking questions; I would have preferred if there were less silent pauses and for the consultation to be more fluent.

The PALS tutor then asked Mr X for his opinions. He thought that I took a detailed history of the pain, noting his weight loss and worries about the signs and symptoms. The feedback was largely positive. Then he said that he had noticed something and asked whether he could share it with the rest of the group. I agreed to this, since I believed that any critical feedback is beneficial and it may have helped other people in the group. The diagnosis behind this case was pancreatic cancer and he thought that I was laughing inappropriately during the consultation, bearing in mind the patient's emotional state. He thought that it may have been because of an artificial setting and suggested that I should approach each opportunity as if it was a real situation.

I was nodding to his comments as he spoke, but many thoughts were going through my head. I remember the exact point when I laughed; when he was communicating about his weight loss, he chuckled and said that he was not complaining about it. In my opinion it sounded like a joke, so I thought it was reasonable to acknowledge it. However, was I laughing unconsciously to disguise my nervousness? Was I laughing during those pauses to fill in the awkward silence? I was unsure.

I was not upset with regards to what happened, but I did feel that I could justify what Mr X thought was inappropriate. I decided to accept the comments. Nonetheless, each consultation is a learning opportunity. However, my viewpoint changed as a re-thought the situation. I imagined that the consultation was exactly the same, the only difference was that Mr X was a real patient I was asked to clerk in the GP practice. In this situation, even if the patient felt uncomfortable about my non-verbal communication, he would probably not inform me. Mr X only shared his thoughts because it was a teaching session. Therefore, even if I was capable of justifying myself, it would not have altered the outcomes.

I have always recognised the importance of non-verbal communication skills. They are necessary in establishing a rapport with the patient and thus, may facilitate the process of history taking. This event allowed me to understand that when dealing with sensitive patients, care must be taken not only with what you say, but also with what you do. In this circumstance, it was a patient who was worried about his unexplained weight loss, and I could have made him more comfortable by showing more empathy. I have also learnt to appreciate things I do well, as opposed to constantly criticising myself. Consequently, I can continue to do things that facilitate a process and make subtle improvements where needed.

**PLEASE COMMENT ON THE REFLECTIVE AND ENGLISH
COMPONENTS OF THIS ESSAY:**

COMMENTS ON REFLECTION

This is a good example of true reflection. The author uses the pronoun "I", expressing clearly how he felt before, during and after taking the history, after the feedback from the patient, and then reflects after the event. He clearly found this a useful and memorable professional learning experience, discovering how easily a fine line can be crossed. The consultation is a crucial part of the doctor–patient interaction and in many ways more difficult to teach and learn than a practical procedure. A good consultation is the foundation of the doctor–patient relationship.

The essay could have been even better had the author provided a little more detail about the "patient" and the history and whether he thought at the time that the patient truly was laughing or cracking a joke about his weight loss. It is very difficult for the reader to get a feel for the atmosphere in the consulting room and whether the patient was generally very serious and sombre about himself and his condition throughout, in which case unprompted humour might have been inappropriate, or whether this was a more light-hearted "role-playing" consultation, in which case the student's reaction might have been in tune with the patient's presentation and mood. How upset, if at all, was the "patient"?

Patients usually want their doctor to be human, sensitive, compassionate and, perhaps most important, interested. Laughing with a patient is not bad practice, but has to be done carefully, sensitively and appropriately. Humour can be very therapeutic if the dose, frequency and timing of administration are carefully judged. Doctors who laugh with their patients would usually be perceived as being on the same wavelength. Doctors who do not pick up on a patient's humour, refuse to join in or distance themselves could be considered by patients and their relatives as cold, aloof, uncaring and disinterested. It could be argued that the author was being a little too self-critical but he accepted the "patient's" opinion (which for the purposes of this interaction was the only one that mattered), did not defend his laughing and simply analysed his reactions.

Non-verbal communication, eye contact, facial expressions and body language, which the author also touches on, are also important. Sadly, nowadays, doctors often hide behind a computer screen, "fenced off" from patients, but this can be mitigated by sensible organisation of the consulting room furniture.

COMMENTS ON ENGLISH

What was done well

➤ The essay is well paragraphed; each segment of the story falls into its own paragraph, making it very easy for the reader to track the sequence of events.
➤ The essay also contains many effective sentences that vary in length and structure to add pace and meaning to the writing. The following extract is particularly effective: "I was not upset with regards to what happened, but I did feel that I could justify what Mr X thought was inappropriate. I decided to accept the comments. Nonetheless, each consultation is a learning

opportunity." The longer sentence is followed by a shorter, powerful sentence, which is then followed by a longer sentence. Vary your sentence length. It is a simple and effective way of adding meaning and style to your writing.

The extract would perhaps read better if rewritten as:

I was not upset when the patient criticised what he thought was inappropriate laughing, but which I thought I could justify. I accepted his comments. I am aware that there is something to learn from every consultation.

What could have been done better
➤ The author generally uses full stops appropriately but his grasp of the comma is less secure. Use commas to indicate where you would like or where you think the reader should pause to capture the meaning of the phrase, or to separate a clause from the rest of the sentence (*see* Chapter 2). The following extracts use commas inappropriately and could be improved by removing them altogether:

1 We were already taught the structure of a history, and this session was based on practical clinical scenarios.
2 I was nodding to his comments as he spoke, but many thoughts were going through my head.
3 In this circumstance, it was a patient who was worried about his unexplained weight loss, and I could have made him more comfortable by showing more empathy.

These examples show the student using commas before or after a connective. The words "and", "but" and "because" are all connectives and are used, unsurprisingly, to connect two clauses in a sentence. Generally, you do not need to use commas around a connective.

Index